KU-689-732

Contents

Part 3 Increasing the credibility of the message: peers and patients as health promoters

P/O NO:
ACCESSION NO: KHO2364
SHELFMARK: 616.9792/AiD

Part 4 Gaining the support of those with influence   65

Preface

This book is intended primarily for health promotion planners and educators dealing with the spread of acquired immunodeficiency syndrome (AIDS) in their countries. It examines one particular aspect of the AIDS pandemic: the reaction of individuals and groups to AIDS, and how health promotion programmes can take these reactions—which are often irrational from a public health point of view—into account.

The idea for this publication came from discussions with colleagues working in AIDS control, who pointed to major problems in their efforts to design information and education programmes about AIDS. They perceived a need for more insight into some of the sensitive issues surrounding AIDS, such as the denial by certain groups of the extent of the problem, the reluctance of decision-makers to admit that "unacceptable" sexual behaviour exists, the difficulties encountered in designing effective messages without offending religious beliefs and moral convictions, the social taboos that discourage open discussion about sexual behaviour, and the extreme fear experienced by some at low risk of AIDS who over-react and call for isolation of infected people.

Following these discussions, it seemed useful to search for examples of how others have faced the problems caused by reactions to the AIDS pandemic: reactions of denial, fear and blame, often retreating behind social mores and taboos. This publication presents case studies of this nature. It is divided into four sections. Part 1 focuses on the health promoters themselves: how they can deal with their own emotions and reactions to AIDS and AIDS education. Part 2 focuses on target audiences: how their emotional responses to AIDS can be used to increase the effectiveness of educational messages. Part 3 illustrates how patients and peer groups can motivate others to change risk behaviour, while Part 4 focuses on decision-makers and "gatekeepers", who can help or hinder health promotion, and examines how their support can be enlisted.

Although many of the case studies are based on experience in industrialized countries, where the epidemic first came to public attention, they are not without relevance to developing countries. The growing body of experience in developing countries now being recorded should, as it is published, provide a most useful complementary source of information and lessons learnt.

This collection of case studies is the product of collaboration between WHO and the Royal Tropical Institute in Amsterdam, Netherlands. The contributions of Riet Berkvens and Maeve Moynihan of the Royal Tropical Institute are gratefully acknowledged.

PART 1
Starting with ourselves

This section looks at the strong emotional influences experienced by health promoters in dealing with HIV and AIDS. Maeve Moynihan poses a number of questions that could be asked to illustrate how emotions can influence the professional judgement of health workers. Hilary Dixon and Jane Springham take the exercise further. From their experience of training professionals to respond more effectively to AIDS, they are aware of the strong emotional reactions that may emerge in response to the concepts of death, promiscuity, anger, sexuality and pain. They provide examples of how confused or unrecognized values and feelings can impede education, and they offer practical suggestions for overcoming those barriers.

Emotional responses to the AIDS pandemic

Maeve Moynihan[a]

The current situation

As the problem of acquired immunodeficiency syndrome (AIDS) affects more and more countries and greater numbers of people, provision of information and education has become a major weapon against the disease, and a way of encouraging appropriate reactions to it.

One of the lessons to emerge from the health promotion programmes that have been functioning for some years is that, at each stage of planning and implementation, decision-making tends to be affected by the emotions that AIDS arouses. Each programme has its own reactions to contend with as well as those generated by the press, by government announcements, and by the many interest groups within the community. Examples of decision-making that seems to be governed more by feeling than by thinking can be found at almost every level of society.

At the government level, examples can be found in decisions concerning the testing of visitors for the human immunodeficiency virus (HIV). Several national authorities require visiting students from some countries to be tested for HIV antibodies, but not students from others. Elsewhere, HIV antibody tests are required for new immigrants, but tourists, businessmen and diplomats are usually granted exemption. Elsewhere, decision-makers may attempt to minimize the extent of the domestic AIDS problem for fear of reducing the inflow of tourists. It is difficult, from a public health perspective, to see how these different measures can lead to reduction in the spread of HIV. The decisions seem rooted in an assessment of the political impact of interest-group reactions and popular sentiment rather than in considerations of public welfare.

There are also numerous examples of over-reaction among health professionals. In one country a group of senior nurses have refused to do thick blood smear tests for malaria. Elsewhere, nurses have refused to care for

[a]   Health Educator, Royal Tropical Institute, Amsterdam, Netherlands.

dying AIDS patients. Both groups know that their duties do not put them at risk if they observe simple precautions, but knowledge is not enough; their fear is so great that it prevents them from acting rationally.

Similar examples can be found at the community level. People who are at little risk may have an exaggerated fear of acquiring HIV infection, insisting on the imposition of rules tantamount to punishment for infected people. In one country, a schoolgirl who contracted HIV through a blood transfusion was enclosed in a glass box while she was at school. In another, a man dying of AIDS could not sell his car, because potential buyers were afraid of infection; the man was also asked to stay at home and not mix with his neighbours.

Fear gives rise to a need to apportion blame. In some countries blame has often been attached to homosexuals. Indeed, AIDS has sometimes been portrayed as happening only to white homosexual males. The people who insist on viewing AIDS in this way often claim to be at no personal risk at all.

People who engage in high-risk behaviour often use the same defence mechanisms. In some countries, men do not consider themselves to be homosexual if they have sex with women as well as with men. By identifying the same group—white, male, and homosexual—as the people to blame, others can deny that the disease has anything to do with them. They may even avoid seeking information about AIDS for fear that their self-image will be threatened.

This combination of denial and blame has been found to operate among decision-makers also. Certain community leaders have claimed that their communities are completely risk-free (and by implication, blame-free) and have stopped all discussion of sexual behaviour in general and AIDS in particular. Similar patterns of denial and avoidance have been found among some communities of prostitutes (Schoepf, 1988).

These brief examples of the way people have reacted in different cultures cannot indicate the great complexity and variation of the reactions. Each country, and each group and person in the country, develops an individual approach to the disease, depending not only on the numbers of patients and spread of the disease, but also on reactions and adaptations to it. In addition, the situation in any given country is continually changing.

However unique it may seem, AIDS is not completely different from other public health problems. Brandt (1988), writing on the history of sexually transmitted diseases (STDs) and the lessons they might have for those working with AIDS, made four important points:

- The emotion that the disease arouses has influenced and will continue to influence medical approaches and public health policy.
- Promotional activities that attempt to stop undesirable sexual behaviour on the basis of fear alone do not work. However, those that combine a judicious amount of fear with a practical way of modifying high-risk sexual behaviour (which in STD control usually means promoting the use of condoms) can have some success.
- Compulsory testing, *cordons sanitaires,* and other similar measures are not effective.
- Even when treatments and vaccines become available, they will not easily modify or end the pandemic.

These points have a direct bearing upon the subject of this publication, and indicate the path that health policy-makers must take. Health promotion activities are of central importance to efforts to prevent and control AIDS. If the right approaches and policies are to be adopted, professionals must somehow learn how to handle strong emotions that may be only half-consciously recognized.

Reactions of health professionals

It may be thought that the professional judgement of health workers is never clouded by emotion. One way to gauge this is to ask the questions listed below—recognizing that the area is one where there are few right answers—and monitor the person's emotional reactions.

The health workers should be asked to imagine that they are visiting a hospital outpatient clinic and see two mothers with babies; one baby has measles, the other has AIDS, acquired from the mother, who is HIV-infected.

- What is their first response to the two mothers? Is it the same for both?
- What if the mother was infected with HIV by a blood transfusion rather than by sexual contact? Does their attitude to her change?
- Will they put more effort into treating the baby with measles because

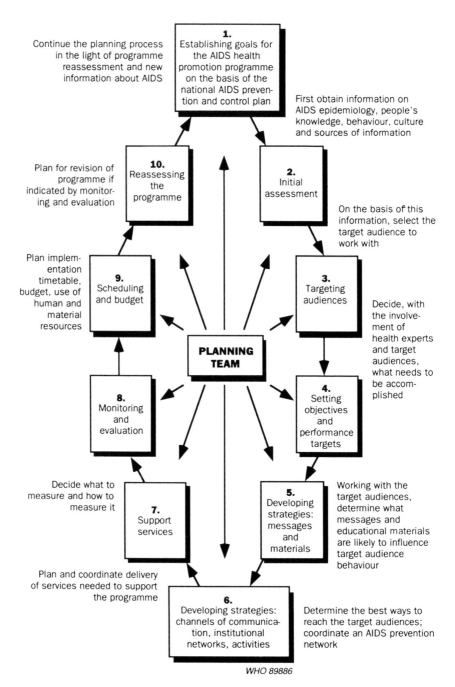

Continue the planning process in the light of programme reassessment and new information about AIDS

1. Establishing goals for the AIDS health promotion programme on the basis of the national AIDS prevention and control plan

First obtain information on AIDS epidemiology, people's knowledge, behaviour, culture and sources of information

Plan for revision of programme if indicated by monitoring and evaluation

10. Reassessing the programme

2. Initial assessment

On the basis of this information, select the target audience to work with

Plan implementation timetable, budget, use of human and material resources

9. Scheduling and budget

PLANNING TEAM

3. Targeting audiences

Decide, with the involvement of health experts and target audiences, what needs to be accomplished

8. Monitoring and evaluation

4. Setting objectives and performance targets

Decide what to measure and how to measure it

7. Support services

5. Developing strategies: messages and materials

Working with the target audiences, determine what messages and educational materials are likely to influence target audience behaviour

Plan and coordinate delivery of services needed to support the programme

6. Developing strategies: channels of communication, institutional networks, activities

Determine the best ways to reach the target audiences; coordinate an AIDS prevention network

WHO 89886

Fig. 1. Elements of planning for health promotion

he/she will live? Is there very little that can be done for the baby with AIDS? Will they become frustrated by spending time and effort on a child who will die?

- What about the mother who is HIV-infected? Would they have delivered her baby?
- Do they think that there is any possibility that they might be infected? How do they feel about their own death?

Next, the health workers should be asked to imagine that they have been asked by a voluntary organization to talk about AIDS to a group of teenagers who have dropped out of school.

- Do they know the common words used in the street for the male and female genitalia, for different sexual activities, and for condoms? Do they feel at ease using those words in situations where they are necessary for instruction? Can they discuss such things with their children or with their partners? Are they at ease demonstrating how to use condoms to a group of the opposite sex?

Finally, they should imagine that their AIDS programme has limited funds and they have to consider requests for support from three organizations—one working with people with haemophilia, one with homosexuals, and one with drug injectors.

- What are their criteria for setting priorities? Do they feel that one group has more moral worth?

The health workers should then consider whether answering these questions has provoked any feelings in them? Have they spotted issues that are sensitive for them? Most people would say yes; if health promoters admit to being influenced by their emotions, then it is worth while asking when and where this occurs. In the health promotion planning cycle (see Fig. 1), the health professionals' own objectivity and ability to learn might be most affected at step 2, the initial assessment, when information is obtained on AIDS epidemiology, people's knowledge, behaviour, culture, and environment, and at step 5, when strategies, messages and educational material are developed. As the cycle continues, the emotional reactions of the target audiences themselves come into play (WHO, 1989).

References

Brandt, A. M. (1988) AIDS in historical perspective: four lessons from the history of sexually transmitted diseases. *American journal of public health,* **78**(4): 367-371.

Schoepf, B. G. (1988) *Community-based risk reduction support*. Paper presented at the First International Symposium on Education and Communication on AIDS, Ixtapa, Mexico, 1988.

WHO (1989) *Guide to planning health promotion for AIDS prevention and control*. Geneva, World Health Organization, 1989 (WHO AIDS Series 5).

Overcoming barriers in ourselves

Hilary Dixon[a] and Jane Springham[b]

What are the barriers?

Death	Sex	Isolation
Dying	Illness	Bereavement
Prejudice	Discrimination	Risk
Disfigurement	Dependence	Loss of employment
Sexism	Prostitution	Promiscuity
Anger	Pain	Conflict
Disability	Uncertainty	Racism
Drugs	Despair	Fear

In our experience of health promotion against AIDS, issues such as those listed above are likely to be raised in some form or another. For most people, merely reading the list probably conjures up emotive pictures or elicits an instinctive response.

Some of the subjects are taboo and rarely talked about even within an intimate relationship. Some elicit uncomfortable feelings we may prefer to avoid. Still others are associated with recollections from childhood, such as the way we were touched and spoken to, the atmosphere at home, the family, the physical environment, school, our peers, our religion. Our feelings about them have been shaped by the values and attitudes to which we were exposed when we were young, and gradually modified as we have gained experience ourselves. The values and attitudes of those around us were in their turn shaped by the whole range of religious, moral, legal, ethical, and social mores of the society in which we live. All of us bring these feelings, values, and attitudes into our relations with others, and what we say and do are greatly influenced by them.

In our professional lives, we cannot simply set aside this complex web of feelings, values, and attitudes for the duration of the working day, picking

[a] Team Manager, AIDS Education Unit, Cambridge Health Authority, Cambridge, England.
[b] Director, Cambridge AIDS Programme, Cambridge Health Authority, Cambridge, England.

it up again when we go home. The planning that is essential to the success of any work must therefore include some personal preparation. This involves becoming aware of the areas and issues that are difficult for us, beginning to work on them, and identifying support for dealing with them. If we do not do this, our own feelings, values, and attitudes are likely to become entangled with those of the people with whom we are trying to work. This will certainly create confusion and may entirely negate the value of any work we do.

It is important also to recognize that the people we work with have their own feelings, values and attitudes. If we hope to bring about any change we will need to acknowledge this, feel at ease with emotions, and develop the skills to handle them appropriately.

This preparation is necessary for all forms of health promotion against AIDS whether we are providing information, examining feelings, values and attitudes, or developing skills.

Providing information

The information we give and the way we present it are value-laden. Decisions such as the weight to give to conventional medical treatment as opposed to holistic approaches, the emphasis to give to condom use, or how to mention oral and anal sex are all influenced by our personal value systems. Health workers employed by an agency that specifies clearly what may or may not be said in health promotion will have to censor certain information and have other information specifically approved.

We need to monitor the way we present information and be aware of the reasons for presenting it in the way we do. To what extent are we influenced by external factors, about which we can often do little? To what extent are we influenced by internal controls we impose on ourselves or by personal opinions? Two examples may help to illustrate this situation.

■ Betty is a teacher. She feels uncomfortable with the issues raised by HIV infection and AIDS, but they are part of the syllabus and she is required to teach them. In talking to her pupils, Betty explains about the high-risk behaviour practised by many prostitutes, intravenous drug users and homosexual men. The young people get the impression that AIDS has nothing to do with them. Betty is saved the embarrassment of any difficult questions.

■ Martin has been invited to provide a training session for volunteers on an AIDS helpline. They are discussing sexual activity in terms of high, medium or low risk. He suggests that anal sex is much more risky than vaginal sex. One of the group challenges this and asks for the evidence. Martin feels uncomfortable; he is not sure what the evidence is, he just "knows" that it is true. Afterwards, he wonders why he felt so uncomfortable. Was it just because somebody had challenged him or had it to do with his belief that anal sex is dirty and unnatural?

Both Betty and Martin were uncomfortable about an aspect of what they were talking about. If they had prepared themselves both professionally and personally they might have handled the information very differently. Betty might have understood how important it is in health promotion not to isolate young people from the very real problems that may affect them. Martin might have checked his information and recognized that, in this case, his beliefs happened to be factually correct. However, beliefs often get in the way of evidence. He could usefully have discussed this phenomenon with the group.

In presenting information we need to ask ourselves four questions:

- **Why am I presenting this information?**
  This will enable us to clarify objectives for a particular group. For some groups only the most basic information is necessary about the nature of the disease, the transmission of the virus, and methods of protection. For other groups it may be necessary to discuss specific concerns, such as occupational risk or drug injecting.

- **What do I want the group to get from the information?**
  Some groups, such as young people, need to understand that the information is of direct relevance to them. In other cases, it may be more appropriate to reassure the group that the likelihood of their becoming infected is very small. The way the information is presented will determine its effect.

- **How can I best present the information?**
  Each group responds differently, and consideration needs to be given to the most effective method of presentation—lecture, quiz, video, or question-and-answer session.

- **Am I at ease in communicating this information?**
  If we experience any discomfort or find ourselves censoring our responses to any of the above three questions, we have some prepar-

atory work to do. Discomfort about any of the information will certainly be transmitted to those listening. If we censor certain information we are influencing the quality of the education given to the group.

Examining feelings, values, and attitudes

In working on issues related to AIDS, we need to go beyond mere information. Most educators now recognize that feelings, values, and attitudes must be taken into consideration in encouraging change in behaviour and providing sensitive care for people infected with HIV.

To help others explore their feelings, values, and attitudes, it is essential to remain objective, to empathize without becoming emotionally involved, to listen with respect, and to challenge where necessary. This is not always easy, and thorough preparation, support, and external supervision are necessary. Practical experience also helps in approaching a group with confidence.

> ■ Peter is exploring attitudes towards homosexuality with a group, and they have just seen a video tape that looks at society through the eyes of a homosexual. One of the group rushes from the room in tears. Some of the group want to go and find the person, others accuse Peter of being insensitive since he does not go himself.

> ■ Jenny is just coming to the end of a training session for first-aiders when one of the group says that none of the information he has been given will change his opinion, he would not give first aid to a drug addict or a homosexual. The group turns on him to demand an explanation, to question what he says, and to ridicule his attitude. Jenny has ten minutes left to deal with this situation.

Both these situations are difficult to handle. Peter is probably right not to go and find the person, who may well be thinking only of himself or herself by leaving a session that was in some way painful. At a suitable break he may inquire about the person and offer to listen if he or she wants to talk. Very often the person will be ready to rejoin the group. However, Peter will also need to talk to the group and reach agreement to continue.

If Jenny is to be an effective health promoter she will need to challenge the statement that has been made, while acknowledging the fear underlying it. At the same time she will need to deal with negative responses from the rest of the group. If Peter and Jenny are thoroughly prepared they will be aware of the difficulties that may arise, will have talked about various ways of handling them, and may well have observed other trainers in the same situation. They will then feel less threatened when difficulties arise.

Groups can be extraordinarily reluctant to look at emotional issues and may use a wide range of avoidance techniques. Health promoters need to be aware of this avoidance behaviour and have the confidence to confront it when it arises.

■ Ann is running a session with a group of medical students on attitudes towards HIV infection and AIDS, and holding a quiz on transmission of the virus. She is attempting to make the discussion personal, and to focus on the group's own perception of risk-taking. The more she tries to do so, the more the students want categorical answers about what is and what is not risky. Finally, one of them says, "Look, all we want to know is whether we are at risk from patients."

■ Tony is working with a group of young offenders. Somebody asks where the virus originated. The group quickly lapses into speculation, anecdote, and media-inspired stories. In a short while, they are looking for scapegoats and blaming others for what has happened. They all feel better now that they do not have to take any personal responsibility.

■ Sheila is running a two-day course for health visitors. She gradually becomes aware that the group does not regard AIDS as a problem that affects them. There is an implicit assumption, which everyone appears to have adopted, that as educated, married, sexually faithful, law-abiding citizens none of them is at risk and that the problem is one that affects only uneducated, unmarried, promiscuous, irresponsible individuals.

In all these situations the group became uncomfortable with the subject under discussion. If Ann, Tony, and Sheila permit the group to distance itself from the issues they will not be carrying out effective health promotion. They need to confront the situation by describing what they observe, suggesting why it is happening, and asking the group to reflect on whether this is a useful approach. They are more likely to recognize what has happened and have the confidence to challenge it if they have themselves been part of a similar group.

Developing skills

Our own feelings, values, and attitudes also influence any skill training we offer. We may need to work with groups on decision-making, communication, negotiation and assertiveness skills, or on practical skills such as how to use a condom effectively. Groups may also need to practise how to communicate these skills to others. If we lack confidence or feel uncomfortable with any of these skills, it will show in the way we teach them or avoid teaching them. As educators we must be able to help others to overcome fear and embarrassment.

> ■ Pam is an AIDS trainer and has just completed a series of sessions for workers in a drug rehabilitation centre. She talked about the important role condoms play in the prevention of HIV infection, handed out leaflets about condoms, and left some sample packets on the table for people to look at. When she made a follow-up visit to one of the drug centres, she was surprised to find that no-one was demonstrating effective use of condoms to the clients. With much embarrassment, one of the workers admitted that he did not know how to demonstrate their use, and another said she had never actually handled a condom.

> ■ Chris was working with a group of social workers who were considering their own attitudes towards HIV infection and AIDS. They several times raised the issue of assertiveness. One woman said she would find it very difficult to negotiate with a man what kind of a relationship she wanted with him, and this met with general agreement. Chris did not follow this up; she knew she was not very assertive herself, and these social workers seemed very confident to her. She thought that they might recognize her own lack of assertiveness.

In the first example it was clearly not enough for Pam to lecture or to distribute leaflets and condom samples. The group needed to talk about their own anxieties, ask questions, gain confidence, and handle condoms. In the second example Chris did not take up the issue of assertiveness because she lacked confidence herself. In both cases the educators needed an opportunity beforehand to deal with their own anxieties and embarrassment.

Overcoming barriers in ourselves

It is relatively easy to recognize that there are barriers, both in ourselves and in those we instruct; it is much more difficult to overcome them. How do we prepare ourselves personally for AIDS health promotion and at the same time establish support and supervision?

Preparation

The most valuable preparation is to form a resource group with fellow workers. These may be colleagues in the same organization or like-minded people in a similar field. Such a group has three useful functions.

- It provides a forum for discussing methods and materials. It can assess the usefulness of material produced locally, nationally, or even internationally. Group members can be encouraged to bring material they have produced themselves. The creativity of the group can be used to devise new methods and materials. A simple resource—a picture, for example—can be developed in many different ways into a story, a play, a puppet show, or a discussion.

- It provides an opportunity for testing methods and materials. A good working principle is never to use any method, material, or exercise that you have not tried out yourself; you may not realize how powerful or disturbing the experience can be. Testing activities with colleagues also leads to useful discussion about presentation skills, the value of the activity, and the way in which it is carried out.

- It provides an opportunity for discussing sensitive issues in a supportive environment. By taking part in the group's activities you may become aware of what you yourself find hard to deal with and so be alerted to potential difficulties. It may be appropriate to deal with such issues together with the whole group or with a single partner. In the latter case you may find listening techniques useful. In conversations we often do not register all the information being given because we are preoccupied with preparing our response. Equally, when we are talking we may speak quickly for fear of being interrupted, or avoid a sensitive issue in case the discussion becomes emotionally difficult. Practising listening to a partner for five or ten minutes without interrupting or judging can help you hear and absorb what is being said, and ensure that the other person has the opportunity to explore an issue in depth.

Sometimes you may not want to use such a group for personal exploration; you may want to take time alone to reflect on aspects of your own life or on an issue that has created difficulties for you. Occasionally you may need more help than the group can offer. If so you might consider consulting a professional counsellor or a medical or health professional.

Support

Clearly the resource group can continue to offer support throughout the health promotion programme against AIDS. However, there are additional ways you can seek support once you start work.

● It can be a valuable experience to work with a partner. This allows tasks and expertise to be shared and provides support. When something goes badly it is useful to have someone with whom to commiserate, to analyse what went wrong, why it went wrong, and what you could do differently next time. On the other hand, your partner can praise and encourage you when things go well.

● Monitoring and evaluation of the health promotion programme can provide useful information. Opportunities for participants to reflect and discuss in pairs or as a group help them to assess what they have learnt and how they are responding. However, you will probably also need to use formal evaluation techniques. Pre-test and post-test questionnaires designed to measure changes in knowledge, attitudes, and behaviour are useful. In an area subject to rapid change, it is important to monitor constantly the suitability of what you are doing. It is very easy to become complacent and continue to deliver the programme that worked well last year but may not be suitable this year.

You are unlikely to be able to influence greatly the support given by your supervisors, but if you have responsibility for other staff it is important to recognize the need to support them. Providing services for people with HIV infection or AIDS, and for their friends, lovers, and families, is stressful; the atmosphere is often emotionally charged and resources may be in short supply. Health workers can lose sight of their own needs in an effort to make things easier for their clients. Regular informal staff meetings are essential for good communication between all levels. Managers need to arrange supervision sessions with individual staff in which difficulties can be identified and stress dealt with before it escalates. They also have a responsibility to ensure that staff have sufficient free time.

It is clear that all this is no easy task. All of us learn through our mistakes, and only through action can we gain experience and become more effective. If we have prepared ourselves thoroughly, both personally and professionally, and have adequate support and supervision, we have at least begun to demolish the barriers to effective health promotion against AIDS.

Approaching your audience: emotive appeal, tone, and setting of messages

Part 1 discussed the emotional reactions of health workers to HIV infection and AIDS. The four articles in this second part focus on the community and target groups for health promotion, discussing how emotion may affect individuals' reactions.

William Smith and Mary Debus describe the thinking processes of a fictional woman called Marie, an 18-year-old prostitute in a large Latin American city. She hears a radio spot on AIDS as she prepares to go out, and her possible feelings, attitudes and responses are explored as they affect her decision on whether or not to pay attention to the message. This leads to a discussion of the kind of information that needs to be collected if health promotion is to be effective for women like Marie, and of how that information can be obtained.

Jon Baggaley examines health promotion programmes for the control of sexually transmitted diseases between the First and Second World Wars and the major lessons learnt. He reviews studies of health promotion for cancer control and the results of a study on AIDS that demonstrates how tone of voice, appeal to emotions, and wording can influence the effectiveness of health promotion messages communicated via the mass media.

Margaret Winn describes a health promotion campaign against AIDS developed in Australia, which used a frightening television advertisement of the scythe-bearing symbol of death knocking over human skittles. It was enormously successful in creating awareness about AIDS, but it also created a huge demand for information—mainly from low-risk groups—for which the health services were not prepared.

Michael Helquist and Godfrey Sealy give an account of a play about AIDS written and produced in the Caribbean area. The use of theatre provided an excellent context for the presentation and discussion of difficult issues and emotions.

The role of qualitative research in AIDS prevention[a]

William A. Smith[b] and Mary Debus[c]

Marie, with whom we begin this paper, is in fact a figment of our imagination. Marie is 18 years old and lives in a large Latin American city. She is unmarried and the mother of a two-year-old daughter named Consuelo. Marie is a prostitute, a professional sex worker.

We first meet Marie at home, preparing for her nightly sojourn in a local bar. As she leaves for work, a radio announcement catches her attention; it says simply "The Government announced today that 50% of local prostitutes are infected with the AIDS virus." Marie stops for a moment, looks towards her dressing table where she keeps a supply of condoms, and leaves for work, having decided that tonight she will not take any condoms along.

Marie knows the basic facts about AIDS. She knows that condoms can provide some protection, and after the radio announcement she even knows that many women like herself, in her own community, are already infected with HIV. Yet she decides for some reason not to use that knowledge tonight to protect herself. Clearly there is a critical gap between Marie's knowledge and her practice.

Our present understanding of AIDS and its impact on people at high risk suggests that three factors may help to explain Marie's decision. First, even though Marie knows about AIDS, she may not feel that she is at risk. In study after study, we continue to find people who know about AIDS and are at risk saying things like, "AIDS? No, not me, it won't happen to me", or "Who knows if AIDS really exists anyway?"

A second hypothesis to explain Marie's behaviour is that she does not think that AIDS is as serious as other problems in her life. The loss of her

[a] Written under the auspices of the AIDSCOM project, funded by the United States Agency for International Development.
[b] Executive Vice-President, Academy for Educational Development, Washington, DC, USA.
[c] Senior Vice-President, Porter Novelli, Washington, DC, USA.

livelihood, inability to support her daughter, her self-esteem may be more important to Marie than even the threat of death. Death seems remote and distant to Marie, not sufficiently substantial to present a real threat.

A third explanation centres on Marie's unwillingness to insist on condoms. Marie may feel at risk and may even take AIDS seriously; but if she does not like or trust condoms she may fail to protect herself.

Those are three of many possible explanations for Marie's behaviour. But each explanation leads towards quite different educational efforts:

— to personalize the risks of AIDS;

— to dramatize the deadly consequences; or

— to improve the image of condoms.

What specific educational intervention will be effective for Marie and other women like her in this particular community? Qualitative research can help us to answer this question and to understand the gap between knowledge and practice that leaves these women unprotected. We might begin our research by asking Marie some qualitative questions, not through a survey but perhaps in a focus-group meeting or in an in-depth interview, or as part of an ethnographic study already taking place in the local community. We might use a sentence-completion technique, with questions such as: "When I think about AIDS, the thing I worry about most is . . . "

In qualitative research the response categories are rarely predetermined, and Marie's first answer might be followed by a series of probing questions, such as:

● Why do you feel that?

● Does this happen often?

● Can you think of other reactions you've had in the past?

We might decide to use projective techniques, for example, showing the photographs of two couples (opposite), and asking: "Which of these couples do you think will use a condom tonight?" This could be followed by probes such as:

● Why do you think so?

● Tell me more about that couple.

● What about the other couple?

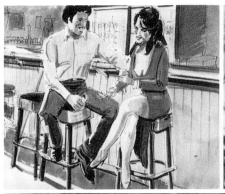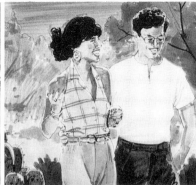

"Which of these couples will use a condom tonight?"

Or we might choose a "ladder technique", in which a series of questions moves Marie backwards or forwards in time from a key event, as steps in a ladder. This may help us to understand better how Marie perceives the event and its relationship to other important aspects of her life. For example, we might begin by asking: "Marie, what would happen if you got AIDS?" Marie's first answer could be "I might die", and we could follow with questions such as, "What would happen just before you die?", and then, "What would happen to your friends? To your family? To your daughter?"

The ladder technique can be particularly useful in establishing links that are not immediately obvious to outsiders. There are, however, many other qualitative techniques to help explore why Marie has failed to protect herself.

What might we learn from this qualitative research process? First, Marie may mention her daughter Consuelo over and over again: "My daughter, she's the only thing that's really mine." "Consuelo would be alone." "What would happen to Consuelo if I got AIDS?"

We might also find that when we showed Marie the pictures she was very definite in saying that one couple would use condoms, since the other couple looked like steady partners who had been together for several months; she may even have remarked that "lovers don't need condoms".

Thus we learn from our research that Marie fears AIDS, but worries more about her daughter than herself. She trusts condoms, but does not think condoms are necessary with a steady partner. In fact, the reason Marie did not take a condom along that particular night was because she planned to be with a man she has known for over three months. Marie told herself that her steady lover could not be infected with HIV.

Qualitative research can help us understand feelings, values, attitudes, prejudices, and fears. The questions are open-ended, often followed by probing questions such as "Why?", "Why not?", "Under what circumstances?" Many questions are likely to arise as the interview proceeds, to follow unexpected leads. One objective is to find links between ideas that are not immediately apparent. To Marie, fear, love, abandonment, and daughter are linked, with her daughter as the central element in her world. This understanding gives us, as educators, an effective starting-point for an educational strategy.

Qualitative research can be vital in understanding why people fail to act even though they have both knowledge and understanding. However, despite its importance, qualitative research is often seen as superficial and hopelessly biased or, alternatively, as a quick answer to all research needs.

The first point of view has some validity. Like anything else, qualitative research may be poorly executed. To be effective, it must be rigorously designed and carried out by experienced professionals. This means, for example, that people in focus groups should be homogeneous and be selected to reflect precisely the group to be studied. Interviewers must be experienced in putting people at ease, using group dynamics, asking open-ended questions without biasing the answers, and developing probing questions that follow the group's thought processes.

Data analysis is frankly subjective. Data are not summarized as "percentage of respondents who . . . ", but rather as themes that recur—ideas that may explain why someone feels at risk or denies being at personal risk. By maintaining quality standards, we can ensure that qualitative research is neither superficial nor biased. Each technique has rigorous standards which must be understood and respected. We must then recognize that not every conversation is an in-depth interview, not every group meeting a focus group, not every village visit an ethnographical study.

The second view is equally dangerous. Qualitative research can be seductive. Because it uses a small number of respondents, it can be done quickly, and because it does not require extensive computer analysis, it seems like a quick and practical alternative to survey research. It is not. Qualitative research, even when executed perfectly, is not sufficient in itself to guide most of our programmes.

Many of the most effective research programmes today combine qualitative and quantitative methods. They use focus groups and ethnography to develop hypotheses, and survey research to validate the results for large-scale populations. One critical role for qualitative research is to put the A in KABP (knowledge, attitude, behaviour, practices) studies, to ensure that our understanding of the gap between knowledge and practice is based on an awareness of how people feel about themselves, about their relationship to AIDS, and about the available alternatives for prevention. Once the emotional elements in the situation have been charted, they can be taken into account. Qualitative research is no panacea, but, if carefully and rigorously executed, it can be a vital part of programme planning.

Media health campaigns: not just what you say, but the way you say it

Jon Baggaley[a]

Past experience with public health campaigns suggests that the mass media in isolation have little effect on health-related behaviour and have to be combined with other elements for a campaign to be successful. They can, however, be effective in increasing public awareness. A number of countries have reacted to AIDS by developing campaigns using the mass media, particularly television and film, to convey messages that generate strong emotions in the viewer. This article deals with the role of mass media campaigns in health promotion and, in particular, Canadian research into the perceived effectiveness and potential side-effects of AIDS campaign techniques.

A seventy-year-old tradition

In 1921 film was in its infancy. However, it was already apparent that the new medium held great promise for the mass communication of facts about health. Agencies concerned with the prevention of sexually trans-mitted disease were particularly enthusiastic about it. Yet their plans for the public distribution of films dealing with sex education met with strong opposition.

Psychiatric and medical opinion was opposed to the public use of films for sex education, on the grounds that they would either give offence or unwittingly condone sexual irresponsibility by tending "to break down the sense of reserve, modesty, or shame" (Lashley & Watson, 1921). The need for greater public awareness of sexually transmitted diseases was less in question than the explicit manner in which commercial films on the topic attempted to generate such awareness. The controversy, in short, bears a striking resemblance to the 1980s debate on the use of the mass media for AIDS prevention.

---

[a] Professor of Education, Concordia University, Montreal, Quebec, Canada.

The dilemma was tackled in 1921 in an exhaustive study by the noted psychologists Lashley and Watson. After interviews and questionnaires covering 4800 people, they concluded that hard facts presented in a serious straightforward scientific manner were unlikely to harm anyone. Certain other techniques, however, were liable to have less desirable effects. Gratuitous dramatization and storyline techniques were considered particularly risky, since they "hold attention more through their action than through their relation to [the facts]". The use of popular colloquial terminology was also criticized as tending to diminish a campaign's scientific credibility.

Lashley & Watson also pointed out that young people tended to respond to sex education defensively, with "flippancy and innuendo", while with other audiences "the danger of arousing disturbing fears is a serious one". They saw a straightforward expository approach as the only way in which these contrasting negative reactions could be avoided.

Has anyone tested these conclusions in developing public education programmes about AIDS? Apparently not. Since 1986, AIDS campaigns have run the gamut from hard-sell dramatic techniques, such as those used in Australia and the United Kingdom, to the soft-sell, even light-hearted, approach of several Scandinavian campaigns. This range of strategies has been particularly apparent in the contrasting campaigns waged through television, with the widest of all audiences (Baggaley, 1988a).

Has human nature therefore changed since 1921, becoming more amenable to health promotions in all its forms? Numerous studies suggest that this is not so. The resistance of prime target audiences to educational campaigns has been noted with such consistency that by now one would have thought that something would have been done about it—that campaign planners would have agreed on the most productive approaches.

The literature on AIDS education to date indicates no such action, no such agreement. The consensus of educational research has remained remarkably consistent in encouraging the straightforward expository approach in media campaigning, as opposed to the more eye-catching, dramatic approach. However, as Hyman & Sheatsley (1947) pointed out, such evidence seems "often to be overlooked in the general eagerness simply to distribute more information". Mendelsohn (1976) suggests that "[much] of what we see in so-called mass education in public health today is more often designed to please the whims of some well-meaning board members than it is to accomplish meaningful effects." Or in Hindson's words (1985), most media campaigns are "little more than short-term propaganda exercises . . . having little impact on the world's major health problems".

Obstacles to effective media campaigns

A major obstacle to media campaigns appears to be the failure of public health agencies and education departments to collaborate in the campaign planning process. As Job (1988) points out, "the final say in mass media campaigns is often given to bureaucrats who do not have a working knowledge of the principles of behavior change." Lacking any media skills whatever, health agencies typically delegate the sensitive task of campaign design to media advertising agencies, though, as Job argues, "there is good reason not to expect a strong parallel between health promotion and commercial advertising [techniques]".

Advertising agencies, though highly skilled in attracting public attention to a new product or social issue, are conspicuously less successful in creating new psychological needs or altering old ones. Moreover, their traditional research methods—despite an assiduously cultivated myth—are surprisingly inadequate for the task of identifying effective propaganda techniques. Their techniques, favouring eye-catching dramatization and popular forms of language, are precisely those considered by Lashley & Watson in 1921 as likely to trivialize a health campaign and decrease its credibility. In the context of AIDS education, the predictions of Lashley & Watson about the potentially undesirable effects of ill-designed public sex education may already be becoming true.

Many of the initial AIDS awareness campaigns in a number of countries were evaluated in 1988. The general outcome of those campaigns has been an increase in public awareness of the AIDS problem, but failure to change AIDS-related life-styles other than in certain high-risk communities where the campaigning has been intensive and carefully concerted. In particular the resistance of young people to AIDS information has become painfully apparent (King, 1988).

This chequered experience with the mass media has led health promoters to a somewhat reactionary view of the media's value as campaign tools. In this view, use of the mass media has little effect on health-related behaviour and must be combined with other approaches for a public health campaign to be successful. However, if media campaigns did not continually contradict and conflict with one another, it is at least arguable that their effects would be more substantial.

Comparison of media campaign styles

A rare opportunity to study the impact of health promotion through the media arose in 1981, thanks to the Canadian Cancer Society (CCS). Public education about cancer risks and cancer prevention is of central importance to the CCS, which has spent many millions of dollars on educational campaigns using local and national media. However, it began to fear that its conventional campaign approaches were failing to communicate with a major sector of the Canadian public—the "functionally illiterate" members of society (i.e. those with less than a full high-school education), who are at the greatest risk of cancer.

To investigate this, the CCS commissioned an evaluation of a selection of its most widely used smoking prevention campaigns. The study was conducted between 1981 and 1985 at universities in Newfoundland and Montreal, under the direction of the present author (Baggaley, 1982, 1986a, 1986b, 1986c, 1987). It emerged that typical smoking prevention campaigns were indeed ineffective.

Readability tests indicated that printed material destined for the public was often unintelligible to people with less than a college education. Billboard campaigns were either disregarded or simply not noticed. Campaign material in general—even the most expensive film and television productions—was as likely to increase viewers' resistance to giving up smoking as to reduce it.

The CCS sought to overcome these problems by attempting to determine which campaign techniques were most effective among different types of audience. The major obstacle to media campaigns proved to be not so much public illiteracy as the psychological resistance of audiences at high risk. The study then focused on the ways such resistance might be anticipated and overcome.

A wide range of survey techniques were employed, from the questionnaire and interview methods of conventional programme evaluations to a series of innovative research methods associated with the media advertising industry, the latter including moment-by-moment analyses of audience responses to media techniques (continual response measurement (CRM)). Multivariate statistical analysis was also employed in the effort to identify the effects of media techniques upon specific audiences.

The research indicated that highly defensive high-risk audiences (e.g. smokers) may reject a media programme on the slightest pretext. A particular turn of phrase or momentary loss of interest can generate negative attitudes that persist for the remainder of the programme and beyond. Such audiences were particularly critical of attempts at dramatic characterization and of the realism or relevance of dramatic situations. They suspected all but the plainest of statistical evidence and were apt to detect a preaching or patronizing approach where none could conceivably have been intended. In one situation, an actress portraying a doctor was judged to be unbelievable because her performance was too polished.

In a purely negative sense, the studies indicated the need for greater sensitivity in the selection of words, visual images, and even vocal inflection in efforts to overcome the audience's defences. More positively, they indicated constructive ways in which defences could be overcome. Even high-risk viewers reacted positively to preventive advice that acknowledged the difficulties of modifying high-risk behaviour, and they invariably welcomed practical tips that might be helpful for that purpose. They proved amenable to scientific authority and to subtle suggestions that their behaviour might be harmful to family or friends. These findings furnished practical hints to the designers of anti-cancer campaigns on how to overcome the types of resistance their productions might encounter.

Putting research into practice

In another study, a film on skin cancer was evaluated. A sample of rural fishermen—particularly older men accustomed to stripping to the waist in the sun's full glare—showed intense resistance to the idea of using preventive filter creams. They readily accepted that filter creams were effective and that their sons should be encouraged to use them, but they seemed reluctant to use them themselves. This observation was immediately utilized by the director of a CCS film on skin cancer, who inserted a sequence in which a young fisherman was shown using a filter cream while his father watched. On the film's soundtrack the father cautiously approved the son's behaviour. When the film's effect was judged after-wards, the older men's apparent resistance to filter creams was found to have been completely overcome.

The director of the film showing the female doctor character who had been criticized as being too polished responded to the finding by retraining the actress to speak her part in an apparently boring monotone. Though surprised, she did so and was subsequently judged by a sample of the target audience to be totally believable, an obviously authentic doctor. This course of action would not have become apparent without the second-by-second precision of the computer-based CRM methods em-ployed in the study. (It should be noted that advertising researchers are currently using these methods with increasing enthusiasm in the pilot-testing of commercials for beer and hamburgers.)

It is worth noting as well that, in both the CCS cancer study and the AIDS prevention studies, this technique produced results that consistently sup-port Lashley & Watson's conclusions on the merits of straightforward campaign styles, the frequent pitfalls of the more elaborate dramatization techniques, and the often defensive attitude of young people towards health education.

Side-effects of AIDS education through the media

In 1988, the research team involved in the CCS studies compared televised public service announcements (PSAs) about AIDS by measuring audience reactions to them in Canada, Norway, Sweden, the United Kingdom and the United States of America. The comparison revealed a wide range of production approaches and a correspondingly wide range of audience responses.

As in the previous studies, the campaign programmes perceived by viewers as the most effective from an educational standpoint were those that presented hard facts in a simple and straightforward manner. Com-plex and emotional techniques elicited negative responses. Light humour was accepted by high-risk viewers, though it was concluded that it might well produce less favourable reactions if it was not used carefully. One observation in this study was that the announcements judged to be the most successful by the sample (high-risk and low-risk viewers alike) had not been sanctioned for general broadcast, usually owing to their explicit-ness. The announcements that had gained the widest public exposure were those our viewers judged to have the least educational potential, being cautious and vague.

Audience reactions to AIDS prevention campaigns, as measured in this manner, were found to be significantly related to their effects on knowledge and attitudes. The campaigns were observed to have affected the sense of urgency with which subjects regarded AIDS as well as their tolerance towards people with the disease. These results support findings by other writers (Fineberg, 1988a, 1988b; Wober, 1988). For example, it was found in 1986 that Canadian television viewers with a high risk of contracting HIV infection were more liberal than low-risk viewers in their attitudes to AIDS-related civil rights issues. They were also more knowledgeable on AIDS issues generally. Although the film material used in this study has since received widespread international approval for its effectiveness in increasing public awareness of AIDS, high-risk viewers in the study reacted to it in a markedly defensive way. The attitudes of high-risk and low-risk viewers on AIDS-related issues were found to have diverged dramatically following exposure to the film.

As measured by questionnaire, the programme evidently increased the sensitivity of high-risk viewers to AIDS-related civil rights issues. It failed to alter the relatively intolerant attitudes of low-risk viewers to those issues. Attitudes of high-risk and low-risk viewers towards the urgency of AIDS as a social issue also appeared to have polarized; high-risk viewers exhibited a relatively low sense of the urgency of AIDS issues, low-risk viewers an increasingly high sense.

In general, it was concluded that an otherwise useful film had unwittingly polarized viewers' responses on psychological measures of fundamental social importance. The polarization was assumed to be attributable to the common instinct of viewers to seek to protect their individual rights on the basis of their assessment of their own AIDS risk (Baggaley, 1988b, 1990). The perceived low urgency on the part of high-risk viewers was attributed to a denial reaction.

These studies indicate that, when seeking to increase knowledge of AIDS without adequately catering for effects on fear and tolerance, educational strategies may be directly responsible for psychological "boomerang" effects opposite to those intended. Even the best educational material so far available may generate such effects because of the extreme defensiveness of high-risk recipients.

The need to be sensitive to AIDS campaign style

Our most recent analyses establish a direct connection between the unintended boomerang effects and specific momentary reactions to the educational material, as measured by CRM methods. These results underline the need to be sensitive to AIDS campaign styles. As with the corresponding samples in our previous studies, high-risk viewers appear to be prone to judge an educational programme negatively on the basis of the slightest momentary shortcoming, e.g., a brief digression to explain something they already know, an unnecessary visual illustration, or a graph they can dismiss as ambiguous. Multivariate analysis and causal modelling techniques show their responses at such moments to be significantly related to their overall reduced feeling of urgency about AIDS and their increasing self-protectiveness in relation to tolerance.

Such effects support Job's conclusions on the nature of adverse public reactions to anti-smoking and road safety campaigns (Job, 1988). Even tenuous evidence, Job indicates, can lead "to quasi-logical support for the denial type of response [by high-risk audiences] which alleviates any existing fear". This response leads to the assumption that "the health promotion campaign is wrong or I am special and immune in some way (e.g. a very good driver)". Obviously such reactions are unjustified on any reasonable grounds, but they should none the less be forestalled.

Our current studies demonstrate that unintended effects of this sort can easily be avoided by simple alterations to educational films at the post-production editing level, and that such improvements may rapidly be overtaken as old facts, methods and terminologies become outdated.

For the present, however, we remain confident that careful testing of educational strategies by up-to-date programme evaluation methods will generally lead to the development of more efficient approaches to AIDS prevention. We believe that, on this basis, a more effective role will be found for the mass media in AIDS education and that growing awareness of the psychological responses to public campaigning techniques will lead to a consensus among educators, policy-makers, and the community members concerned regarding the most acceptable educational approaches.

References

Baggaley, J. P. (1982) Electronic analysis of communication. *Media in education and development,* **15**: 70-73.

Baggaley, J. P. (1986a) Developing a televised health campaign: I. Smoking prevention. *Media in education and development,* **19**: 43-47.

Baggaley, J. P. (1986b) Developing a televised health campaign: II. Skin cancer prevention. *Media in education and development,* **19**: 86-90.

Baggaley, J. P. (1986c) Formative evaluation of educational television. *Canadian journal of educational communication,* **15**: 29-34.

Baggaley, J. P. (1987) Continual response measurement; design and validation. *Canadian journal of educational communication,* **16**: 217-238.

Baggaley, J. P. (1988a) Perceived effectiveness of international AIDS campaigns. *Health education research,* **3**: 7-17.

Baggaley, J. P. (1988b) Campaigning against AIDS; a perspective for Southern Africa. *Media in education and development,* **21**: 106-109.

Baggaley, J. P. et al. (1990) AIDS education: the boomerang effect. *Studies in educational evaluation,* **16**: 41-62.

Fineberg, H. V. (1988a) Education to prevent AIDS: prospects and obstacles. *Science,* **239**: 592-596.

Fineberg, H. V. (1988b) The social dimensions of AIDS. *Scientific American,* **259**: 128-134.

Hindson, P. (1985) IUHE President's message to the World Health Education Conference. *Irish medical times,* **19**: 25.

Hyman, C. F. & Sheatsley, P. (1947) Some reasons why information campaigns fail. *Public opinion quarterly,* **11**: 413-423.

Job, R. F. S. (1988) Effective and ineffective use of fear in health promotion campaigns. *American journal of public health,* **78**: 163-167.

King, A. (1988) *Report on national survey on Canadian youth and AIDS.* Ottawa, Canada, Department of Health and Welfare.

Lashley, K. & Watson, J. (1921) A psychological study of motion pictures in relation to venereal disease. *Social hygiene,* **7**: 181-219.

Mendelsohn, H. (1976) Mass communication and cancer control. In: Cullen, J. et al., ed. *Cancer: the behavioral dimensions.* New York, Raven Press.

Wober, M. (1988) Informing the British public about AIDS. *Health education research,* **3**: 19-24.

The Grim Reaper: Australia's first mass media AIDS education campaign

Margaret Winn[a]

Background

After the deaths from AIDS of a number of babies in 1984, the Australian Federal Government took the lead in the campaign against the disease. It successfully mobilized bipartisan support for its policies, ensuring a cooperative countrywide effort in the fight against AIDS. Federal coordination of the national response, among other things, permitted:

- the endorsement by State health ministers of a national health strategy for AIDS control;

- the development of a uniform policy on blood donation;

- the introduction of universal HIV antibody testing of donated blood and blood products;

- the establishment of various advisory committees with representatives from a wide range of disciplines and parties;

- the development of a national education strategy for AIDS.

These initiatives provided a solid foundation of public confidence in the Government's ability to respond appropriately to the AIDS threat and set the stage for a public campaign.

The national education strategy aimed to furnish education and support for community groups seen to be at high risk of HIV infection. However, the risk of spread of the virus to the heterosexual population, highlighted at the Second International Conference in Paris in June 1986, convinced government advisers of the need to extend the campaign to the wider public. At the beginning many Australians had seen AIDS as a disease confined to homosexuals. However, as the number of AIDS cases reached epidemic proportions, high-risk sexual behaviour and needle-sharing

a   AIDS Bureau, New South Wales Department of Health, Sydney, New South Wales, Australia.

were seen to be widespread in the general community. Thus, when the Government embarked on a national education campaign, the principal objective was to make HIV/AIDS a matter of concern and relevance to all Australians. The mass media were chosen as the channel to disseminate the message quickly and persuasively.

The campaign was preceded by carefully managed promotion. In order to maximize its impact, great secrecy surrounded the content.

The campaign

The campaign was launched dramatically in April 1987 as a week of prime-time television spots. It featured the traditional symbol of death, the Grim Reaper, as a scythe-carrying skeleton in mediaeval garb, who night after night bowled over human skittles in an underworld bowling alley. No one—baby, child, man, or woman—was spared the merciless assault.

It had been intended that the television spots should encourage people to seek further information, so in the following months additional advertisements were placed in newspapers, cinemas, and magazines and on the radio. The follow-up material emphasized prevention and contained comprehensive information about transmission, safer sex, and the antibody test, as well as contact numbers for further advice.

The campaign message was a blood-chilling one: the HIV/AIDS epidemic is advancing remorselessly, it is an inescapable part of our lives, we are all potentially at risk, prevention is the only cure. It was a message to make people sit up and pay attention. And they did. Almost immediately everyone seemed to be talking about AIDS, everyone had a view, the topic was discussed at every dinner party.

Successes

Unquestionably the campaign was enormously successful in creating awareness of AIDS. An unprecedented 97% of those surveyed had seen the Grim Reaper television spots. The campaign disseminated messages about AIDS transmission and prevention to millions of people in a very short period of time, and put AIDS in the forefront of the public mind.

After eight weeks a mid-campaign evaluation was undertaken to compare people's knowledge, attitudes, and behaviour with research data from before the campaign. The principal findings were that misconceptions about casual transmission were less prevalent and attitudes to preventive measures, such as use of condoms and the distribution of needles and syringes, more liberal.

People believed that the Grim Reaper had not only increased awareness and knowledge about AIDS but had also changed people's behaviour.[a]

Many people felt that the campaign had prompted a desire for more information. It certainly created intense public debate. Articles about the relative risks of anal and vaginal intercourse as modes of transmission appeared daily. Discussion about heterosexual anal intercourse, attitudes to condoms, and bisexual husbands was explicit and very public.

By making AIDS a topic for public discussion the television campaign assisted in "the radical acceptance of the previously unacceptable". Programmes broadcast in 1988 about drug injectors, explicit billboard messages on safer sex, and young women promoting condoms on television would have been unthinkable before the campaign.

By opening for public examination subjects that the churches had traditionally seen as their concern, the campaign prodded them into becoming involved in AIDS programmes and in a range of subjects from condom use to care for the dying.

Sexually transmitted disease clinics reported a significant change in attitudes to condoms. In the commercial sex industry, brothel managers and, to a lesser extent, clients no longer actively discouraged condom use and many establishments supported sex workers who wanted to use them.

There had been unarticulated support for direct and explicit education prior to the Grim Reaper campaign, but after the campaign questions were raised about the lack of comprehensive school education on AIDS. The state departments of education were given a clear mandate to proceed with the inclusion of education on HIV/AIDS in the school system.

After the campaign, corporations and community groups of all kinds began to see a role for themselves in AIDS prevention and control, and a chance of funding. This resulted in a proliferation of organizations

---

[a]   That is, other people's behaviour, although 44% claimed it had changed their own behaviour.

providing AIDS-related services and a bureaucracy to support them. The growth of this AIDS industry was accompanied by a wide variety of approaches and activities, and this diversity, coupled with the public debate and resultant increase in knowledge, has been a positive outcome of the campaign.

Less welcome results

The Government wanted all Australians to see AIDS as being of personal concern to them. However, the Grim Reaper campaign did more than that: for many people, it created unnecessary fear and, often, great anxiety about their past behaviour.

After the first television spots, laboratories performing HIV antibody tests were swamped with work. There were huge increases in the number of heterosexual men and women attending clinics and ringing telephone information services. These men and women did not, as the campaign had intended, want more information about AIDS. In fact, at the major AIDS clinic there was no increase in the number of requests for general information about symptoms, transmission, or safer sexual practices. Rather, people wanted to be tested, to allay the fear that their past behaviour had resulted in infection. The Grim Reaper campaign induced a large number of low-risk people to seek not information but reassurance. This obviously raises questions about the value of inundating services with unjustifiably frightened low-risk people.

In contrast to low-risk heterosexuals, there was no increase in the number of homosexual men or male and female prostitutes attending clinics. At the major AIDS clinic there was even a drop in the number of homosexual men attending for the first time.

The Government was insistent on providing follow-up information for the duration of the campaign and had enlarged state telephone information services to cope with inquiries. However, the early secrecy surrounding the content of the campaign meant that the services were unfamiliar with the material and unprepared for the overwhelming demand. In addition, supporting literature was not effectively distributed. If all the ser-vices—state, federal, governmental, nongovernmental—had been in-volved, education and counselling resources could have been better integrated with the campaign and fewer people would have been left with the feeling of an inadequate back-up.

Although the mid-campaign evaluation showed no increased prejudice against AIDS sufferers, the reality was somewhat different. The Anti-Discrimination Board recorded an increase in workplace discrimination and harassment and AIDS clinic staff reported an increased feeling of social ostracism among HIV-infected people.

Many AIDS educators, critical of the decision to use an advertising agency to produce health messages, reacted against the campaign's subliminal messages. Many groups had previously worked hard to promote the belief that AIDS is preventable and controllable and that everyone has the power to stop transmission of HIV infection by adopting particular forms of behaviour. The Grim Reaper campaign seemed to undermine that belief by portraying AIDS as indiscriminately and relentlessly eliminating its human victims. As no one had the power to resist, death was inescapable. The notion that people have the means to control their destiny was lost for the sake of a media advertising image. The promotion of the equation "sex = AIDS = death" undermined AIDS prevention work, and the abbreviation "sex = death" raised the spectre of the young generation growing up with inhibitory anxieties about sexual life.

The Government used the fear of death as a trigger to shock Australians out of their ignorance and apathy. Many believe that the exaggerated message had the opposite effect to that intended. Claims were made that the Grim Reaper campaign was merely a strategy to protect the gay community from being blamed for the epidemic. People eventually became bored with the flood of information about AIDS and withdrew from the debate. In some, the overkill merely reinforced their apathy and produced the familiar distancing effect.

Conclusions

At one level the Australian Grim Reaper campaign was an advertising triumph. It not only won an international advertising award, it was also successful in placing AIDS on the national agenda and creating a high level of personal awareness, public involvement, and debate about AIDS.

At another level it was less successful. Australians did not necessarily accept the concept that they were personally at risk. People were frightened, but fear did not necessarily prompt them to seek information about AIDS or about appropriate changes in behaviour. Those at high risk of

AIDS did not seek AIDS services in great numbers, while those at low risk overwhelmed the testing facilities.

Australia has learnt some important lessons from the Grim Reaper campaign. Although the Government considers that it was successful, the campaign will not be repeated. The second phase of AIDS education is less intrusive, less dramatic; it involves targeting of specific groups, more consultation, more participation by the community, and a diversity of educational approaches.

The Grim Reaper campaign has confirmed that advertising and television spots, no matter how powerful, cannot replace community involvement and action.

Further reading

Ballard, J. Politics of AIDS. *Canberra Times*, 14 August 1988.

Harcourt, C. et al. (1988) On the Grim Reaper Campaign. *Medical journal of Australia*, **149**(3): 162-164.

Morlet, A. et al. (1988) The impact of the grim reaper national AIDS education campaign on the Albion Street (AIDS) centre with AIDS hotline. *Medical journal of Australia*, **148**(6): 282-286.

Taylor, W. T. L. (1988) *The grim reaper: the use of research in policy development and public education.* Woden, Department of Community Services and Health.

One of our sons is missing: using theatre to confront sensitive issues

Michael Helquist[a] and Godfrey Sealy[b]

In August 1988, actor Clifford Learmond first played the role of Miguel, a young bisexual man who contracts HIV infection, develops AIDS, and dies, leaving behind distraught parents, a frightened girlfriend, and AIDS-weary friends. The compelling story of how Miguel's family and community cope with the threat and reality of AIDS is the theme of *One of our sons is missing*, the first play about AIDS written and produced in the Caribbean area.

This successful dramatic presentation ran for three weeks in Port-of-Spain, the capital city of Trinidad and Tobago, after which the writer and producer, Godfrey Sealy, developed a plan to take the production to a number of villages in the country. This "village outreach" proposal gained the support of the Trinidad and Tobago Red Cross Society and the Caribbean Epidemiology Centre, and the Norwegian Red Cross Society provided major funding. As a result, the play was staged in 28 villages throughout Trinidad and in two towns on the island of Tobago. More than 3700 people saw an abbreviated version of the play during the autumn and winter of 1988. This international collaboration demonstrated how major donor organizations could work together with local groups to advance both AIDS prevention and community development.

AIDS education through drama

At the conclusion of each performance of the play, the actors were joined on stage by Godfrey Sealy and Ronald John, an AIDS educator and psychologist, who invited questions from the audience. They probed the audience's level of awareness of AIDS and spoke with emphasis about how people can protect themselves from this frightening disease.

[a] Programme Officer, AIDSCOM Project, Academy for Educational Development, Washington, DC, USA.
[b] AIDS educator and playwright, Trinidad and Tobago.

One question that audience members frequently asked Clifford Learmond after the performance was "How does it feel to play the part of someone with AIDS?"

"At first it was difficult for me", said Learmond. "I was sceptical about portraying a young man who gets sick from a disease everyone wants to shun. I worried a little about what friends and the public would think about my playing a bisexual man. But I have come to terms with it. Now I feel very proud to be associated with this effort. I feel that I am doing something important for my country."

Through the dramatic presentation and the follow-up discussion, the actors and educators were able to gauge the public's knowledge of and feelings about AIDS. One of the most striking findings was the significant public confusion about the difference between someone with AIDS and someone who is HIV-infected. While people expected someone with AIDS to be ill, they were less sure about the status of someone who appears to be healthy. This is an important point in a nation where most members of the population do not know their HIV antibody status.

The various audiences also expressed a strong interest in the meaning of the HIV antibody test results. Many wanted to know where they could be tested. Several were worried about being ostracized if they were found to be HIV-infected.

The actors and educators also found that members of the audience, whether urban or rural, posed questions that clearly demonstrated their misconceptions about the transmission of HIV, believing for instance that mosquito bites or kissing would put them at risk of infection. People also wanted to know where they could get more information about AIDS.

Educational material—some prepared specially for the theatrical production—was offered to the audience along with free condoms. People in the villages responded enthusiastically to written material that relied heavily on graphics and picture stories to complement the text.

Specific issues

The production was well received in the villages, partly because it provided live entertainment of a type rarely seen in them, but also because it addressed an issue that had been prominent in the national media in the previous year.

Sealy found that people in the villages were eager to discuss AIDS. Members of the audience were most concerned about the relationships among the characters in the play. Most were sympathetic towards the mother's anguish over her son's illness, and they understood the harsh response of the father to his son. Some said that their attitude towards the son became more sympathetic as the story progressed. Generally audiences were receptive to the idea of support and compassion for people infected with HIV, including those with AIDS, but fear of the disease clearly remains a primary obstacle to personal contact with people with AIDS.

Audiences were generally comfortable with the discussions on sexuality in the play. No one seemed offended by the bisexuality of the main character. The actors found this to be especially true in the villages. John noted that village people seemed more at ease than urban people in talking about sexual issues, the use of condoms, and other safer sex practices. All the men in the village audiences reported on the evaluation forms that were distributed that they were familiar with condom use; the men were also quite pleased to receive free condoms at the end of the play. Women in the audience were more reluctant to take the condoms provided.

John considered that the play provided a way for people to view AIDS in more human terms; AIDS often puts people off or frightens them. One middle-aged woman from the village of Moruga told the actors that when she first heard that the play was about AIDS, she did not want to see it. However, she did see the production, and afterwards commented, "I'm glad I came, I feel much better having seen the play and heard people talk about AIDS. It makes it less scary for me."

Further developments

The actors and production team have joined forces for other dramatic endeavours. They developed a carnival AIDS project and presented a pantomime about AIDS for the free-wheeling carnival in Port-of-Spain in early February 1989. One of the performances of the stage play was videotaped, with support from AIDSCOM, for possible use in training programmes. Other groups have expressed interest in filming the play for distribution in North America and Europe, especially in cities with large West Indian populations.

PART 3

Increasing the credibility of the message: peers and patients as health promoters

Part 2 illustrated the difficulty of making allowance for emotional reactions to AIDS in developing health promotional materials. This section examines one approach to solving many of the problems—the use of peers and patients for health promotion against AIDS.

Roger Staub describes a campaign to reduce high-risk behaviour among homosexuals in Switzerland, in which the chief protagonists were self-proclaimed homosexuals. The campaign led to the development of promotional material—booklets, posters—and a type of condom that met the needs of the target group.

Elizabeth Ngugi and Francis Plummer describe a project in Nairobi, Kenya, that brought together prostitutes to learn the facts about AIDS. The most knowledgeable were then recruited to educate others. One aim of the project was to encourage a large number of prostitutes to insist on condoms, so that clients could not refuse to use them.

John David Dupree and Stephen Beck describe how promotional projects are now using people who are HIV-infected, including those with AIDS, as educators. The physical presence of such people and their comments make educational sessions both more human and more effective. While most of the work is currently being done in the United States of America, the technique is also being tried in Sierra Leone, Uganda, and the Caribbean area.

These papers support the argument that in health promotion pro-grammes on very personal issues, such as sexual behaviour, the person designing and delivering the messages and materials must understand the attitudes of the group being addressed. In terms of understanding and sensitivity, people who belong to the group itself may often be the best health promoters.

The Swiss Hot Rubber Campaign: self-proclaimed gays take responsibility for informing their community

Roger Staub[a]

If the name Switzerland evokes for you images of mountains, cows, yodelling, and chocolate you would not be exactly wrong, but you would miss a large part of Swiss reality. You would be right in thinking of Switzerland as conservative. However, there is a vivid contrast between, on the one hand, the Switzerland of tourist advertising and conservative politics, and on the other the country with one of Europe's highest per capita AIDS rates, an enormous drug problem, and a government with an extremely liberal approach to AIDS.

By March 1991, there were 1778 reported cases of AIDS in Switzerland. The rate of increase in the number of cases in Switzerland is similar to that in the United States of America and Europe as a whole. Switzerland, however, together with France, has the highest per capita rate of AIDS cases in Europe. The rate of HIV infection among male homosexuals is estimated to be between 10% and 20%.

The Swiss AIDS Foundation, established in June 1985 by all the Swiss gay organizations, has played an important role in the initiation of action to prevent HIV infection. Its intention from the start was to combat AIDS in all population groups rather than just among gays. It has become the national umbrella organization for gay groups, drug users, prostitutes, people with haemophilia and others interested in combating AIDS, as well as for the many local AIDS organizations in all Swiss cities.

---

[a] Swiss Federal Office of Public Health, Bern, Switzerland.

The Hot Rubber

By the end of 1984, AIDS and the rumours about it began to cause great alarm, above all in the homosexual community. Certain groups in this community wanted to take swift preventive measures. They began to talk to other homosexuals about condoms, since it was already known that anal intercourse was a major mode of transmission of HIV. Homosexuals had previously perceived no need to use condoms.

The first thing the groups did was to distribute a simple booklet on safer sex, which pointed out the dangers of penetration without protection. To help gays make their choice in what was to them a new area, this advice was accompanied by an advertisement for a well-known brand of condom. The meeting between these two worlds was effected through exchange; the manufacturer paid for the advertisement, not in cash but in condoms, thus enabling 5000 condoms to be distributed with the booklet.

Gays were not very keen on the idea of using condoms. They felt a sort of repugnance for them, having, they thought, consigned them permanently to oblivion. But even though this first experiment was not a great success, it did show the way ahead; it would be useless to try to exploit fear or to ask people to abandon an established practice. The change called for must appear simply as an adaptation, so that it would be widely accepted.

It was thus decided to direct efforts towards a publicity campaign aimed at making the condom familiar and even smart and fashionable. Gays in the advertising profession joined forces with the initial group to help with this campaign. They recommended that information should be supplemented by a marketing campaign based on solid realities. That would mean having the best product, the best design, and as many easily accessible sales outlets as possible. As a back-up to all this there had to be continuous publicity designed to reach all segments of the homosexual population.

Finding the right product required no more than a little common sense. What professional prostitutes used with success could be just as useful for others. So the product existed, but it was of a rather clinical whiteness (Fig. 1). A number of tests had to be conducted to develop a suitable marketing approach. The first attempt failed because the homosexual population did not accept it, but the second achieved very wide acceptance; it had an attractive design and packaging, which did not lend themselves to too many connotative interpretations (Fig. 2). An English name was chosen to cope with the problem of Swiss multilingualism and to appeal to the cosmopolitan attitudes of gays; a trademark was chosen and a distributing firm set up—the Hot Rubber Company, owned by the Swiss AIDS Foundation. In November 1985 the Hot Rubber Company began selling Hot Rubbers in their definitive form at the price of one Swiss franc for two. The entire profits of the company were reinvested in the prevention campaign. Although those who tested the product during its development had not been impressed, when they tried it in its final version they found it finer and safer and the level of sensation high. In a word, they were won over; the Hot Rubber was made for them.

The next step was to bring the product to the people concerned. Bars and saunas, meeting-points for gays, were obvious distribution points. The first stage was to persuade the managers and owners to agree to sell Hot Rubbers in their establishments. After more than two years of effort it is now possible in certain bars to order "a beer with", and be served beer with two condoms. Some saunas make them available free of charge.

Constant efforts are exerted on the publicity front. Every month a new poster comes out, intended for bars and saunas. The regular renewals, adapted to the season of the year and sometimes very amusing, facilitate a wider and more personalized identification with and acceptance of the message and also provide a topic of conversation among the gays. Examples of the many posters produced in the last three years are shown in Fig. 3.

Effects of the campaign

In addition to observations of the reactions of the people concerned, some spot evaluations were carried out. A survey conducted in gay circles in Bern after one year of campaigning asked the question, "What is a Hot Rubber?"; 90% of those polled answered "a condom" or "the gay condom".

The trend of sales figures also speaks for itself (Fig. 4).

The product came on to the market in November 1985. In 1986, 125 000 condoms were sold. The 1987 sales stabilized at around 300 000. This levelling-off of sales may be accounted for by the fact that in the same year the national AIDS information and prevention campaign was getting under way. Major supermarket chains then began to sell products comparable in price and quality with the Hot Rubber. It was at last possible to purchase condoms anonymously, like milk or chocolate.

In summer 1987, the Lausanne Institute for Social and Preventive Medicine, on behalf of the Swiss Federal Office of Public Health, conducted a scientific survey of behavioural changes among homosexuals. Eight hundred questionnaires and 50 personal interviews were evaluated. Most of those questioned were promiscuous homosexuals, and the survey, although not truly representative, can be considered indicative of the real situation.

More than 50% of those questioned lived alone, 25% lived with a partner, and the remaining 20% considered themselves bisexual or were living with a woman.

Some 50% claimed not to have had anal intercourse in the three months preceding the survey; 30% said that they always used condoms during anal intercourse, 20% that they did not. Concerning the last group, it was not determined whether or not the contacts involved steady partners.

Eighty-five percent claimed to have changed their sexual behaviour; 75% said that they bought condoms and 66% stated that they consistently observed the safer sex rules.

On the basis of these data we may assume that one out of five homosexuals continues to be at risk. It is important to note that knowing a person with AIDS was associated with positive behaviour change, but it was not the only factor. We also found that men with many partners, independent of whether they knew anyone with AIDS, adopted safer sex practices more rapidly than other men at risk. It seems that all groups are familiar with the prevention message and appear to follow its rules. In saunas, unsafe sex is rarely practised. In public toilets and parks it is more frequent.

Three problem groups remain:

● Bisexuals often do not think of themselves as homosexuals, and consider that a message addressed to homosexuals does not affect them. They were reached more effectively by the "STOP AIDS" campaigns aimed at the general public.

● Adolescent homosexuals, as they make their first tentative steps into the subculture, are too preoccupied to pay much attention to messages about preventing AIDS.

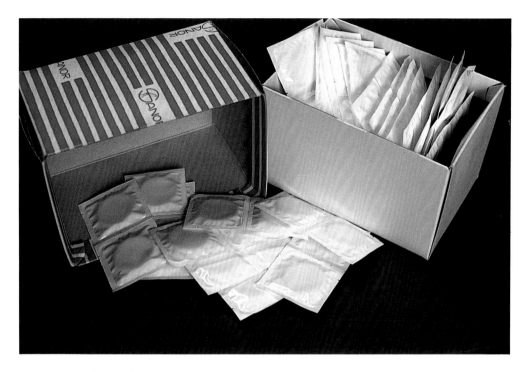

Fig. 1. A condom suitable for use by homosexuals existed – but was of a rather clinical whiteness.

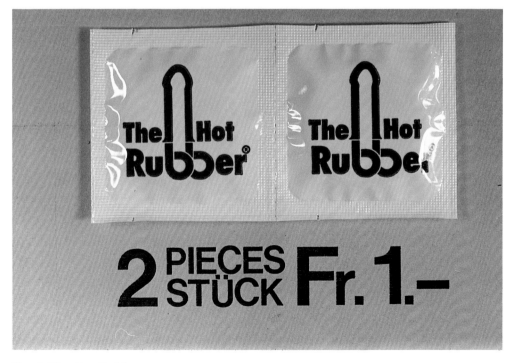

Fig. 2. The Hot Rubber.

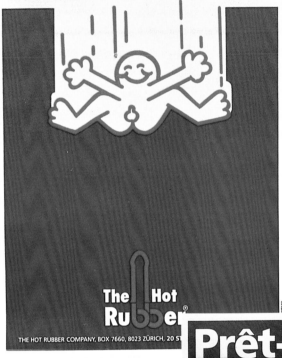

Fig. 3. Some of the posters used to promote the use of condoms among homosexuals.

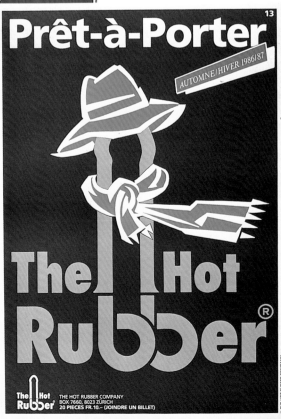

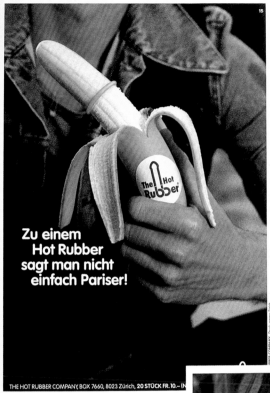

Zu einem
Hot Rubber
sagt man nicht
einfach Pariser!

THE HOT RUBBER COMPANY, BOX 7660, 8023 Zürich, **20 STÜCK FR. 10.–**

Fig. 3. (cont.)

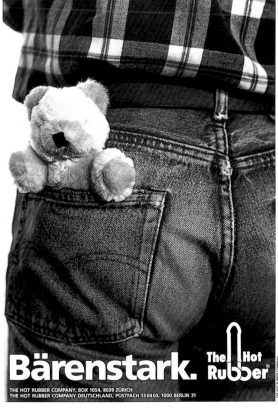

Bärenstark.

THE HOT RUBBER COMPANY, BOX 1054, 8039 ZÜRICH
THE HOT RUBBER COMPANY DEUTSCHLAND, POSTFACH 13 04 03, 1000 BERLIN 31

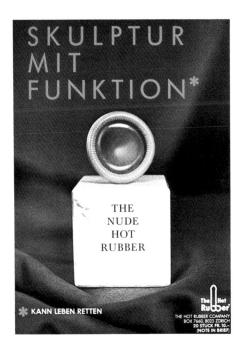

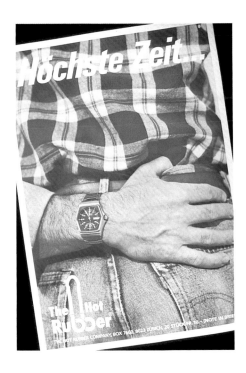

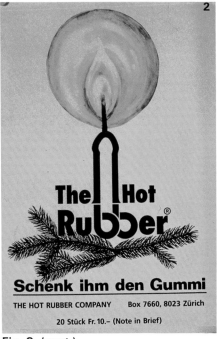

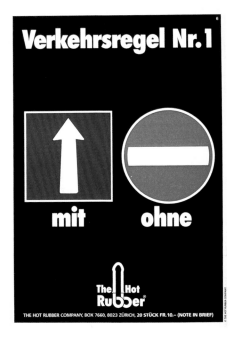

Fig. 3. (cont.)

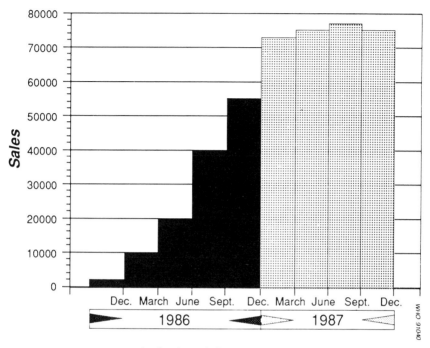

Fig. 4. Trend of sales of the Hot Rubber, 1986–1987.

- Older homosexuals who do not easily find partners are more inclined to dismiss the warning "if it's with me it's with a rubber".

It appears that many gays who find difficulty accepting their homosexuality have problems in changing their sexual behaviour. Prevention efforts should therefore include improving the image of homosexuality and the climate within the gay community. We intend to initiate pilot projects towards this end, specifically targeted at these groups, particularly adolescents and older homosexuals.

Conclusion

The use of the existing structures of an established community—specifically bars and saunas—has certainly been conducive to individual acceptance of responsibility. Thus, instead of being panicked into deserting such places, the gay community has been given an opportunity to change its behaviour. Last but not least, it was self-proclaimed gays who took responsibility for informing their community, and this certainly contributed to the fact that the instructions on safer sex were accepted as preventive and not repressive.

Clearly the campaign has to continue, the object being to increase to 100% within a short time the percentage of condom users among homosexuals in Switzerland who practise anal intercourse. It should, however, be stressed that the Hot Rubber campaign is only part of the preventive work being carried out among that population. It is just one of the Swiss programmes being conducted under the slogan "STOP AIDS".

Prostitutes teaching prostitutes in Nairobi

Elizabeth Ngugi[a] and Francis Plummer[b]

Prostitutes are usually hard to reach. In Kenya, our multidisciplinary health team walked through mud, rain, and hot sun in an effort to meet these women where they live and work and to establish a rapport with them based on mutual trust and confidence.

Before the team started working with the prostitutes towards better health, it was important for the members to go through a "self-awareness" exercise. This enabled them to shed their biases and myths and close the gap between themselves and the prostitutes. Members of the health team asked such questions as:

- How do you manage to work with prostitutes?

- What do you say to them?

- Do you actually sit in the same room with them?

- Aren't you afraid of them?

This calls for an analysis of feelings and attitudes towards prostitutes and prostitution, in order to see the situation without imposing value judgements. Only then can the health worker enter into a useful relationship with the prostitutes that helps them to learn.

The initial contact

How did we find the prostitutes? It is not easy to know who is a prostitute where prostitution is illegal, so we looked at the register of the Skin and Special Treatment Clinic, to which the majority of persons suffering from sexually transmitted diseases are referred. It showed that most of the women and their contacts with such diseases resided in Pumwani. Accordingly we made that area the operational target, following the principle of

[a] Lecturer, Department of Community Health, University of Nairobi, Kenya, and Chairwoman, Health Education Committee, National AIDS Committee.
[b] University of Nairobi, Kenya.

taking services to where the people concerned live and work. We made brief visits to the homes of the women, introducing ourselves as health personnel interested in working with them to reduce the prevalence of sexually transmitted diseases. We approached them as we would any other group of women. We did not call them prostitutes. They told us what they were.

We believe that it was because they understood that we were going to work *with* them, and help them learn how best to reduce the sickness due to sexually transmitted diseases, and that they were going to be active in the process rather than being told what to do or how to behave, that as many as 300 came to the first *baraza* (public meeting). Once we had got to know each other they brought us a wealth of practical knowledge. The fact that they had been accepted as human beings needing support was a tremendous source of motivation for them.

The evolving programme

During the *baraza*, the prostitutes told us what their needs were in relation to the control and prevention of sexually transmitted diseases. There had been no reported cases of AIDS in Kenya at that time. We explained to them how HIV infection is transmitted and what its effects are. We told them how infection could be prevented and invited them to register at a new clinic established specifically to serve them, to distribute condoms, and to provide counselling, diagnosis, and treatment as well as follow up.

The women showed enthusiasm for protecting their own health, and elected a leader and a committee to represent the three villages in which they lived. We trained the committee members in community mobilization and basic communication skills in order to promote condom use. They acted as informal health educators for the rest. We told them that HIV detection and surveillance activities were to commence and invited all the women to take part. The leader was given condoms to distribute to those whose stock ran out between clinic sessions.

The village health committee met the health team every two months, and *barazas* took place every six months. At one of them, attended by about 300 women, we told them that our studies showed that some of them were infected with HIV or with other sexually transmitted diseases. We explained that those who were infected were likely to transmit the infection to their clients, and that those not infected were at risk of becoming infected. The best thing they could do, we told them, was to give up prostitution; the next best was to insist that their clients used condoms.

Educational methods

We used several educational methods. One was a questionnaire testing the women's knowledge of AIDS, of their ability to prevent it, and of how they could teach others to avoid becoming infected. About 250 women completed this questionnaire. The ten giving the best answers were invited to address the other women at the next *baraza* (see Box). They shared with them their knowledge and impressed upon them the nature and consequences of infection with HIV.

Another approach was to use sketches and role-plays reinforcing earlier messages, performed by members of the village committee. A song was also sung by members of the village health committee at a *baraza*.

In addition, group and individual counselling enabled the women to discuss with us their problems and how best to solve them. It emerged during counselling that most of the women wished to change their life-style and give up prostitution. They asked for a rehabilitation programme to train them for other suitable work, as a starting-point for a new life.

Results

The result of these joint efforts was a dramatic increase in condom use. At the beginning, 8% of the women occasionally insisted that their clients use condoms. After a year, more than 50% were making their clients use condoms all the time and a further 40% did so occasionally, with a mean of 72% by mid-July 1988. A small number of women also informed us that they had given up prostitution. These changes, occurring after only a modest educational input, are remarkable since condoms are not readily accepted as a method of contraception in Africa. The outcome of all this was a threefold lower rate of HIV seroconversion among the women insisting on condom use, than among those not insisting on such use.

The ten best replies to the question "How would you teach others to prevent the spread of AIDS?" were as follows:

1. I would teach a group of men and women:
   (a) that they should see a doctor every two months to be examined for sexually transmitted disease;
   (b) that men should use a condom during casual sexual intercourse;
   (c) that all should maintain good personal hygiene by washing with warm water and soap after every sexual encounter;
   (d) that all should wash any towels used to clean their genitalia after intercourse.

2. In order to prevent sexually transmitted diseases:
   (a) women should clean the vulva with warm water after sexual intercourse;
   (b) they should attend a clinic/doctor regularly;
   (c) men must always wear condoms in casual sexual encounters.

3. Sexually transmitted diseases can be prevented by:
   (a) the use of condoms;
   (b) washing with warm water after sexual intercourse;
   (c) taking medication prescribed by the doctor when infected.

4. To prevent sexually transmitted diseases, it is necessary:
   (a) to see a doctor;
   (b) to follow the advice given by the doctor;
   (c) for men to use condoms before engaging in casual sex.

5. It is necessary:
   (a) that men should use condoms;
   (b) that women should go to the doctor/clinic from time to time;
   (c) that they should take medicine as prescribed.

6. It is necessary:
   (a) to teach men to use condoms;
   (b) to see a doctor from time to time;
   (c) to take medicine as prescribed.

7. It is necessary:
   (a) to go to a doctor/clinic immediately when you have a problem;
   (b) to take your sexual contact to the doctor for treatment. If you do not do this, treatment of just one person is useless.

8. It is necessary to require men to use a condom.

9. It is necessary:
   (a) to advise men to use condoms;
   (b) to take preventive medicine.

10. If you know that you are suffering from any sexually transmitted disease, go to the hospital immediately, so that you do not infect other sex partners.

Conclusion

We believe that the main factor that made this programme so successful was the fact that the women themselves were responsible for the programme. This was reinforced by the methods we used: taking services to the people and mobilizing the community. The community responded with a high level of participation, and the prostitutes themselves became the educators of their peers.

Making condoms easily available was another important factor. This depended greatly on the support of the health education services. A third factor was that we succeeded in reaching the clients indirectly through the women, who thus proved to be agents of change for the men.

It is gratifying that even women who were already infected with HIV insisted on the use of condoms. They had been educated to such a level that they appreciated the need to protect their clients.

Because of the encouraging results of this programme there are now plans to train multidisciplinary health teams in four other sites as a preliminary step towards implementing the programme on a national scale.

The role of people with HIV infection, their families and friends as health educators

John David Dupree[a] and Stephen Beck[b]

According to numerous study reports, one of the most significant factors influencing knowledge, attitudes and behaviour in relation to AIDS is acquaintance with someone who is known to be infected with HIV, or with that person's family, friends, and fellow workers. For instance, a study reported at the Third International Conference on AIDS in Washington, DC, in 1987 found that one of the factors significantly associated with adopting low-risk behaviour was the visual image of deterioration of AIDS patients and the impact of the disease on individuals known to the subject (McKusick et al., 1987).

Many people do not acknowledge that AIDS could affect them and their communities until they see the impact of the disease on individuals and their families and friends. Studies in Ghana and Zimbabwe to determine the content of AIDS prevention programmes for Africa indicated that people want first-hand evidence of how people with AIDS look, how they and their loved ones deal with HIV infection, and how society reacts to them (Gordon et al., 1988).

Similarly, one of the most significant predictors of how well people adjust to their own HIV infection is whether they have known someone with HIV (Tross et al., 1987).

Unfortunately, the urgency of AIDS prevention programmes precludes waiting until everybody has a friend or family member with AIDS. By that time it could well be too late for major portions of a generation in some of the hardest-hit areas of the world; many people who could have been saved with timely information on AIDS prevention would have become infected and died.

[a] Programme Officer, AIDSCOM Project, Academy for Educational Development, Washington, DC, USA.
[b] Executive Director, National Association of People with AIDS, Washington, DC, USA.

Early AIDS prevention programmes in Europe and the United States of America took advantage of this personal knowledge factor by applying the "peer educator" model, using people with AIDS, their families, and their friends in public statements and programmes on the disease. The model has been used successfully in other health promotion campaigns. For example, women who have had breast cancer are among the most powerful and convincing advocates of regular self-examination. Similarly, those who have overcome alcohol dependence are effective in providing support for others attempting to do the same.

It followed, then, that teenagers with AIDS might be most effective in reaching high-school students with messages about AIDS prevention, gay men with AIDS in reaching other gay men, black women with AIDS in reaching other black women, and so on. Because HIV does not discriminate on the basis of race, sex, religion, socioeconomic status, sexual orientation, political persuasion, or geographical location, use of people with HIV infection helps combat the stereotyped ideas of who can get this disease.

On many occasions, however, attempts to inform people and combat stereotyping have been thwarted, for example by a resistant school board, an uninformed technical crew at a radio station, or a group of parents afraid of infection. The perceived threat usually dissipates, however, when the objectors are brought face to face with ordinary human beings who have HIV infection.

Evaluations of AIDS prevention workshops consistently show that people are informed and inspired by such encounters. For instance, written comments on workshops conducted in Trinidad and Tobago indicate that the "People with AIDS" panel was one of the most effective sessions on the agenda. Similarly, a 3-hour session on the psychosocial impact of AIDS, at the First National Workshop on AIDS in Freetown, Sierra Leone, with a panel consisting of an HIV-infected Sierra Leonean and a Sierra Leonean who had three friends with AIDS, was evaluated as one of the "most useful" presentations.

The issues involved in implementing this "peer educator" concept in both developed and developing countries can be discussed from the viewpoints of (a) the public; (b) the AIDS prevention programme; (c) the individual with HIV infection; and (d) the spouses, family, friends, fellow workers, and other acquaintances of people with HIV infection.

The public

People with HIV can be among the most effective educators about AIDS. In nearly every society, government officials, educators, community leaders and others have discouraged people with HIV or their loved ones from talking in public about the effects of the disease on their lives. Some of the reasons for this are based on misinformation or stereotyping; others merely camouflage prejudices or "moral" positions. Examples of directly stated or indirectly inferred reasons for resistance include:

- fear of acknowledging that there are people with HIV in the area;

- inability to recognize people with the disease as a potentially valuable resource for prevention activities;

- unrealistic fear of contagion if the infected persons or their carers are in a public place;

- fear of the loss of individual or family privacy;

- fear of the loss of an individual's employment, housing, insurance, or civil rights;

- fear of stigmatization and social rejection of the individual or family;

- fear of violence against the infected person or his or her family;

- fear of "bad press" and/or a loss in tourism or foreign aid if citizens speak publicly about their disease;

- fear that, by spending time on providing education, the person will suffer increased stress and waste energy needed for fighting the disease;

- contempt for the individual, who is perhaps perceived as deserving of the disease and unworthy of public sympathy;

- fear that such public statements will include explicit discussion of taboo subjects, such as drugs, disease, death, sexuality and sexual practices, by people who are not suitable role models.

Some employers have terminated the employment of productive people with HIV because of threats to the business once it is publicly known there is an HIV-infected employee. In addition, families have rejected infected people, churches have excommunicated them, the military have discharged them, and courts have removed their children from their custody. So the decision to admit publicly to HIV infection is not one to be made lightly, or without some protection being guaranteed at the policy-making level.

In many countries the process of making AIDS-related policy decisions has become controversial and emotionally charged. Because AIDS is primarily a sexually transmitted disease, its prevention necessitates talking about taboo subjects like sexuality and specific sexual practices, as well as drug use, disease and death. Defending the rights of a person with HIV infection can be complicated when the person is seen by many as a symbol of aberrant disease-causing behaviour and therefore unworthy of respect—certainly not someone to be invited to speak to children in schools or members of church congregations.

Public fear of this new disease may be accompanied not only by this syndrome of "blaming the victim", but also by the conviction that "it cannot happen to me or my family", since none of "us" do those unspeakable things. The distancing necessary to maintain such a posture is frequently gained at the expense of the individuals or groups of individuals thought to be at highest risk. This inability to see AIDS as a human problem can close the hearts of otherwise compassionate people and prevent them from dealing responsibly with the threat to themselves and their families.

The AIDS prevention programme

Some of the issues faced by public and private agencies involved in AIDS prevention campaigns appear to be virtually universal; others vary from country to country or from village to village. The dissemination of basic medical facts tends to cause less controversy and be less emotionally charged than attempts to deal with specific sexual or psychosocial aspects of the disease.

An HIV-infected individual may sometimes be prohibited from appearing as part of an AIDS prevention programme by, for example, the policy-making board of a school or other institution. When this happens, AIDS educators should continue to lobby and educate the policy-makers and the community to have the policy changed. Interim strategies for such action include:

- "humanizing" the AIDS epidemic by arranging meetings between opponents and proponents of the policy and people with HIV infection and their families and friends;

- inviting the policy-makers to attend talks given to other groups by people with HIV and their families and friends, in as nonthreatening a situation as possible;

- recruiting health care workers and counsellors working with HIV-infected individuals to deliver the sexual and psychosocial messages through story-telling and perhaps some sharing of personal experiences;

- recruiting spouses, family members, friends, and fellow workers of HIV-infected individuals to discuss how the disease has affected them and their loved ones in their daily lives; such people can be very powerful and moving advocates of safe sexual behaviour and the sharing of information on prevention with others.

Ideally, however, the personnel of the programme will need to tailor campaigns to particular groups, using HIV-infected people, their families or their friends, depending on the specific situation. In deciding who would be most effective in a given situation, several factors should be considered, including sex, age, race, socioeconomic status, religion, and political outlook. People are more likely to be motivated to take action if they can identify closely with the presenters. For instance, women with HIV may be more successful in overcoming resistance in a women's group, blacks with AIDS will probably be listened to better by a primarily black audience, young people will pay more attention to another young person with AIDS, and religious groups have been observed to be more moved by hearing the story of people from their own denomination. The fact that people from a similar background as the listeners are affected by the HIV virus also helps counter the dangerously stereotypical view that only certain types of people get AIDS.

When people are recruited or volunteer to act as AIDS educators, it is important that they are made fully aware of, and encouraged to discuss, the potentially negative effects of their participation. While candidates may have already thought about these factors, they should be encouraged to consider in particular the disapproval or rejection that they may encounter, as well as the possible loss of job, family, status, etc.

It is also important that the people organizing the public appearances of infected individuals should maintain as much control as possible over the proceedings. Prior to their presentation, the facilitator might thank the panelists, note that they are taking a personal risk by being there, and strongly suggest that the audience respect the panelists' privacy by maintaining a policy of confidentiality outside the room. While the audience should be encouraged to ask any questions, even embarrassing ones, panelists also need to be free not to answer questions that seem too personal.

Once the panelists have been introduced, the facilitator might suggest that the audience be allowed to ask questions after the panelists have finished their presentations. One effective tactic is for the facilitator to start by asking general exploratory questions of each of the panelists, including variations of the following:

- Can you talk about your life before AIDS? What were your hopes, your dreams? What were your relationships like? What did you do for fun? What were your plans? What did you expect to do with your life?

- People have a wide range of reactions to information about life-threatening illness. Can you describe what your life was like during the weeks before and after you were informed of your own or your loved one's HIV infection or the diagnosis of AIDS?

- Families and friends respond in various ways to the news of life-threatening illness, ranging from total acceptance to total rejection. What has been the reaction of your family and friends to this news? Give both positive and negative reactions, if possible.

- Many adults with HIV infection or AIDS have experienced a loss of identity. They are no longer a social worker, doctor, athlete, mother, or soloist in the church choir, but a person with AIDS. How have you or your loved ones experienced this loss of identity?

- Medical expenses can be devastating, even if a person has a well paid job. What has this been like for you or your loved ones? How have your finances been handled?

- One of the most cruel "punishments" that some parts of our society would inflict on people with HIV is withdrawal of intimacy and sexuality from their lives. Some infected people are even accused of deliberately spreading HIV through unsafe sexual practices. What has been the reaction of your sexual partner(s) to the news of your HIV infection or AIDS? What intimacy is there in your life today?

- You or your loved one has had to face the possibility of premature death. Some people describe themselves as being on a roller coaster of depression, hope, anxiety, denial, exhilaration and despair. Others have embarked on new explorations of their spirituality. Can you describe how you or your loved one is dealing with the possibility of early death?

● Can you talk about your current health status? Are you taking any medications or participating in alternative therapies?

Once the audience starts to ask questions, a vital human bond can be—and frequently is—formed. The instructor of a university-level course on AIDS prevention reported, for instance, that a man who had been openly hostile to and critical about people with AIDS for six weeks in the class appeared to change his opinions dramatically after taking part in a class session with three infected panelists. He approached the instructor afterwards, apologized for his previous behaviour, and obtained a referral to an agency doing volunteer work with people with AIDS. Usually audience members approach the panelists afterwards, thanking them and/or expressing their appreciation through some physical gesture, such as a handshake or a hug.

Face-to-face encounters appear to be extremely effective, since people can take part in a dialogue with the individuals. Members of the USAID-sponsored AIDSCOM project have found, however, that the screening of films can provide an acceptable substitute when personal contact is impossible to arrange. The Ghanaian film, *AIDS: Need for action now*, for instance, which shows a young woman in Accra in the end stages of her disease, has been an effective substitute when local people with HIV are not available. The common thread that binds us as human beings usually motivates people viewing the film to want to help prevent such devastation in their own communities.

People with HIV infection

For people with HIV, deciding whether to admit publicly to the infection is rarely easy. Their health status is a major consideration, since nobody can be expected to make an appearance in public or on film if not feeling well. If the willingness and energy are there, people with HIV form a ready pool of educators able to speak about their experiences, because often they have the time and a deep interest. In addition, studies have consistently indicated that long-term survivors with HIV infection often continue to contribute to society in a meaningful way. The idea that sharing personal experiences can help prevent other people from becoming infected may also contribute to a sense of well-being and a positive self-image, both vital for coping with the disease.

People with HIV commonly became infected through voluntarily taking part in high-risk pursuits. Because of this, they can personify risk and effect. In face-to-face encounters, panelists can give audiences an authentic and comprehensible discussion of risky acts. They may have a good grasp of the language commonly used by people with high-risk behaviour patterns, and of ideas about the most effective prevention messages.

It is important that people's concern about safety and privacy should be respected during their public appearances. Some may want to use pseudonyms, wear a disguise, or prohibit the presence of the media and/or photographers so as to feel secure in a society where harassment and discrimination are common. Since loss of control can be a major issue for people with HIV, it is important that the limits they set should be respected.

If a support group, an association or a clinic is involved in the recruitment and training, and in making arrangements for speakers, scheduling can be more predictable. Because of the vulnerability of HIV-infected individuals to variations in health status, having back-up speakers ensures that scheduled events can go ahead. Having the group evaluate the presentation subsequently provides the speakers with the kind of feedback that makes this activity most worth while for them. If funds are available, speakers frequently appreciate a small payment, particularly those with lower incomes.

Spouses, family, friends, co-workers and acquaintances

Spouses, family members and friends of people with HIV often form groups for mutual support, particularly if they feel that their regular support systems do not provide sufficient assistance. Because of the stigma associated with AIDS, many of the people involved in the care of a person with the disease experience discrimination and rejection. In addition to regular meetings to discuss their feelings and coping mechanisms, groups of such people can share information, deal openly with their emotions, celebrate when celebration is possible, and mourn with other people in similar situations. Holding a party to celebrate the fact that your HIV-infected child will lose the sight in only one eye instead of two, for instance, is something that people uninvolved with AIDS might not understand.

Some members of these groups may decide to educate the public about how AIDS can ravage a family, a church, or a community. Because they so frequently feel alone, many find it therapeutic to share their frustration, anger, joy, sorrow and pain with others by becoming involved as AIDS educators. They, too, must be aware of the potential repercussions of their public involvement in such a sensitive area. Some are embarrassed by the unpredictability of their own emotions and others may be nearly immobilized by grief or by anticipatory sorrow at, for example, the prospect of outliving one's child. Since nearly everybody in the audience is likely to be involved in some kind of family or relationship, they are potentially capable of being touched by such a story, whether or not they have previously felt compassion for people with AIDS.

Revealing the human aspects and emotions involved in the AIDS epidemic is vital in motivating people to take personal, professional and political action, particularly in those parts of the world where the incidence of AIDS is low or not generally known. If individuals or decision-makers can see and meet people who are affected by the epidemic, particularly people with whom they can identify in some way, they are more likely to see the problems as their own.

References

Gordon, G. et al. (1988) Using focus group discussions to generate content and scenarios for an AIDS feature film for African audiences. Paper presented at the First Internatonal Conference on the Global Impact of AIDS, London, March 1988.

McKusick, L. et al. (1987) Prevention of HIV infection among gay and bisexual men: two longitudinal studies. Paper presented at the Third International Conference on AIDS, Washington, DC, June 1987.

Tross, S. et al. (1987) Determinants of current psychiatric disorder in AIDS spectrum patients. Paper presented at the Third International Conference on AIDS, Washington, DC, June 1987.

PART 4

Gaining the support of those with influence

The previous sections have looked at emotions and sensitive issues as they affect health promoters and the communities in which they work, and at how they can be taken into account in health promotion. This final section focuses on individuals and groups who can influence health promotion efforts in a positive or a negative way. A term increasingly used for such individuals is that of "gate-keepers". The papers in this section consider a number of different groups, and discuss how health promoters can work with them as allies.

Graham Collier and Kevin Donnelly draw on the experience of the New South Wales Department of Education in implementing a school education programme. They describe the goals of the programme, which aimed to introduce teaching about AIDS into schools, and list three kinds of groups that were found to influence the process: parents and community groups, religious groups, and special interest groups, such as medical practitioners and people with AIDS. They discuss how a working relationship was developed with these groups, and give information on preparation and teaching within the schools.

Jake Obetsebi-Lamptey describes how people working first on the promotion of family planning, and later on AIDS prevention, realized that progress would be slow and difficult unless all members of the Government were informed and motivated. They decided to make a film for that specific target group, in order to enlist its support.

Introducing AIDS education in schools

Graham Collier[a] and Kevin Donnelly[b]

The global menace of AIDS cannot be overstated. In order to reduce its rate of spread, people everywhere, whatever their cultural or religious perspective, must face the challenge posed by HIV. It is a challenge that requires each of us to reconsider our traditions, morals and values and to respond positively to the pandemic. Rarely is this more evident than when considering the question of how to provide the young people of a community with the knowledge and skills required to help them protect themselves from HIV infection.

Many countries have examined the role of schools in providing education of this type. Schools may or may not be the most appropriate agency, depending on local circumstances. Often, the challenge of providing AIDS education in schools has been too great, because of the sensitive nature of the subject matter.

The basic premise of this report is that high-quality AIDS education is vital and that schools have a primary role in providing it for their students. The paper outlines the steps taken by the New South Wales Department of Education in introducing education on AIDS and sexually transmitted diseases into the secondary school system. The procedure outlined is only one culturally specific approach to the development, implementation, and evaluation of a school AIDS education programme.

The New South Wales Department of Education is directly responsible for the education of approximately 80% of the students in the State. Schooling is compulsory between the ages of 6 and 15 years and the Department has approximately 750 000 students, 48 000 teachers and 2500 individual schools under its charge. Secondary schooling commences at about 12 years of age.

[a] Senior Policy Analyst, AIDS Bureau, New South Wales Department of Health, Sydney, Australia.
[b] Senior Education Officer, New South Wales Department of Education, Sydney, Australia.

The aim of AIDS education in schools

The aim of AIDS education is to reduce the risk of HIV transmission, now and in the future. It is important that the education given should form part of an integrated national AIDS prevention and control strategy designed for that purpose.

While programme goals may vary from system to system, the obvious and overriding goal of a school AIDS education programme is to promote behaviour that prevents the transmission of HIV. It was intended that students completing the New South Wales Programme should be able to:

● understand the nature of AIDS and its transmission;

● make informed decisions about behaviour that protects them from AIDS;

● understand the symptoms of AIDS and seek appropriate medical care when needed;

● value their own health and relationships free from AIDS;

● behave personally and socially in ways that eliminate the risk of spreading HIV infection;

● reject biased information and myths relating to HIV infection;

● develop positive attitudes towards those who are infected with HIV.

To achieve these goals, action was needed to:

● increase the level of knowledge about HIV transmission and AIDS among secondary school students;

● increase the level of knowledge about HIV transmission and AIDS in the community in general;

● increase the level of understanding throughout the community in general, and the secondary school population in particular, of the personal and social problems associated with AIDS and the contributions individuals can make towards reducing those problems;

● increase the interpersonal skills of secondary school students, with particular attention to communication, self-esteem, value clarification, decision-making and relationships.

Ensuring widespread involvement

School education programmes are more likely to succeed if there is consultation with the local community. This is particularly true of programmes that generate an emotional response. Parents and other members of the community involved with the school should be consulted, e.g., religious groups and special interest groups, which may feel that they have a role to play in AIDS education or development of an AIDS programme. In New South Wales, the AIDS education initiatives were carried out with the cooperation of, and funding from, the Department of Health. From the earliest planning stage, the programme was viewed as a joint project.

After the preliminary planning stage, a meeting was held with representatives of all groups and departments involved in, or with a direct interest in, AIDS education. An outline of the proposals was presented and discussion and comments were invited. The association thus established with most groups has been maintained.

Representatives of the two federations of parents' organizations attended the initial meeting and have since remained in contact with officials of the Department of Education. Each time new material is prepared for possible use in schools the parents' representatives are consulted and their suggestions and comments sought. These comments, together with the active support of parents' representatives when the Department's initiatives have been questioned by minority groups or individuals, have been particularly valuable.

The collaboration between the Department of Education and the Catholic Education Office is well established and productive. Informal discussions about the AIDS education programme were held at an early stage and continued throughout the development of the Department's material and the subsequent development of the Catholic Education Office's material. Some of the subsequent criticism from other religious groups might well have been avoided or reduced if their representatives had been involved in the planning and development stages.

Other groups with a special interest in the Department's programme were present at the initial meeting. They included the New South Wales AIDS Council, the Family Planning Association, and representatives of several hospitals offering special AIDS-related services. Some important individuals with a high media profile in relation to AIDS education were also invited to attend.

The New South Wales experience has shown that it is more productive to debate differences of opinion within a small group or committee rather than in the public arena. For that reason it is recommended that all potential opponents of the programme should be represented on planning committees, working parties and other groups.

Consulting the community

In most communities there is likely to be some resistance to teaching about such sensitive areas as AIDS. Early consultation can reduce the extent of resistance and help create a supportive influential group of people prepared to defend the teaching at a later date. Sources of continuing resistance need to be identified and the people involved assured that their concerns are being addressed.

In New South Wales, meetings of parents were held throughout the State, in conjunction with the Department of Health. They provided information about AIDS and the transmission of HIV and created a forum for discussions on AIDS-related issues.

The meetings also gave parents a chance to air their concerns, and those responsible for the programme the opportunity to explain the reasons for the initiatives. The meetings varied greatly from region to region, some being well attended and stormy, others poorly attended and quiet. The success of the meetings depended to a large extent on the skill and experience of those in the chair.

Use of the media seemed to be most successful when the people appearing were considered by the public to be credible, for example church members or parents' representatives.

Developing the AIDS education programme

It is important that AIDS education in schools be aimed particularly at students younger than the age group likely to have risk behaviour. If many students leave school before this age, it may be appropriate to target even younger students. All older students also need to be targeted.

In New South Wales, material was produced for use with secondary school students aged 13–17 years, since this was the group believed to be most at risk (surveys have indicated that up to 50% of these students are sexually active).

Material is currently being prepared for other target groups, including students with sensory and intellectual disabilities and primary school students aged 5–13 years.

The decision on where to place AIDS education in the curriculum is an important one, as the context chosen will provide the framework for decisions about the content, teaching style and teacher.

In New South Wales, it was considered that the programme would be more likely to succeed if presented as a series of lessons within the context of a broader programme dealing with sexually transmitted diseases, sexuality, and human relationships. Teaching sexuality is part of a personal development health education programme that not only provides accurate information about AIDS but also develops student skills in, for example, cultivating self-esteem, communicating effectively, clarifying values, making responsible decisions, and maintaining personal relationships.

It was also considered that, because of the sensitive and controversial nature of the topic, AIDS teaching should ideally be carried out in an environment of good relationships between the teacher and the students and among the students themselves.

Programmes can be developed at the level of the individual, the school, or the education system. Those responsible should have a grasp of the concepts underlying preventive education and of programme development methodology. They should know about HIV infection, be able to prepare programmes that cover knowledge, skills, and attitudes, and be sensitive to the needs and characteristics of teachers and students.

The material produced in New South Wales is a collection of teaching ideas which each individual school adapts according to the specific needs of the students, after appropriate consultation with the community concerned. It includes information about AIDS designed to answer the questions: What is AIDS? How is it transmitted? What are high-risk and low-risk activities, safer sex, safe sex? It also deals with sexually transmitted diseases (STDs): What are STDs? How are STDs transmitted? How can STDs be avoided or the risk of infection lowered?

A series of skill-developing activities are presented, concerned with self-esteem, communication, values, and decisions about sexuality, sexually transmitted diseases in general, and AIDS in particular. The teaching ideas were developed by the Department of Education and tested on selected students and teachers.

Who should teach the programme?

The quality, style of presentation and, ultimately, the impact of an AIDS education programme are influenced by the person who teaches it. Many education authorities consider that such teachers should be specially chosen and trained.

The New South Wales Department of Education has instructed schools to teach AIDS within the context of sexuality, and to teach sexuality within the context of a broader programme such as personal development or health education. In theory, the people who teach those broad subjects have the respect of parents, fellow teachers, and students, wish to be involved, and have the required personal qualities and skills. In reality this is not always the case; when it is not, the quality of the teaching suffers. This is an aspect of the programme that requires urgent attention.

Training of teachers

The training of teachers is vital for the successful implementation of an AIDS education programme. The needs of the teachers should be assessed and appropriate training programmes developed. Well equipped and well trained teachers will have a significant impact on the knowledge, skills, and attitudes of the students in their care.

In New South Wales, individual schools sent two teachers (the principal (or his or her representative) and a teacher of personal development or health education) to attend a one-day familiarization course. Following the familiarization courses in June and July 1987, two-day in-service training courses were conducted for teachers of personal development and health education.

Because the teaching strategies employed in this area are often very different from those used in more traditional areas, there is a constant need for in-service training of teachers, a need made greater by the large turnover of teachers of personal development and health education.

Evaluation of HIV/AIDS education

A special evaluation group was established to monitor the impact and effectiveness of the programme. It contained personnel from the Departments of Education and Health as well as a professional evaluator. The material, the information meetings for parents, and the familiarization courses for teachers were evaluated, and generally considered to have met the needs of the various groups.

Tests of students' knowledge and attitudes before and after the programme were also conducted. The first test indicated a very high level of knowledge about AIDS and its transmission. For that reason, and because the period between the two tests was very short, there was only a small increase in knowledge among the students. The second test indicated a possible shift in attitude from one of blaming certain groups for the disease to acceptance of HIV as a virus threatening everyone's life.

The evaluation results have already assisted greatly in the planning of future initiatives.

Conclusion

Teaching AIDS in schools raises many potentially contentious issues. While the personal, community and global benefits of effective AIDS education are generally acknowledged, the fear of addressing such a sensitive issue sometimes results in failure to act. However, we are convinced that with careful planning and consultation many of the difficulties can be overcome. In relation to AIDS education particularly, school decision-makers must not abrogate their responsibility towards those in their care.

Influencing decision-makers through video: experience in Ghana

Jake Obetsebi-Lamptey[a]

Ghana was the second developing country in the world—after India, with its Nirodh programme—to institute retail services for contraceptives. That was in 1971, when we started to advertise condoms and vaginal foam contraceptives. Up to about 1980, we used radio, television, billboards and point-of-sale advertising for condoms. Then in 1979–80, there was a change of government and problems arose within the family planning programme itself. These difficulties resulted in donors withdrawing their support, and everything seemed to collapse.

In 1985, the Government appointed a Technical Committee on AIDS. The Committee's chairman appeared on radio and television and used the newspapers to spread information about AIDS, but there was insufficient funding for educational campaigns. So the Committee chairman introduced the idea of raising funds from both the public and the private sector.

In 1986, the Ghana National Family Planning Programme launched a new social marketing programme for condoms, foam tablets and oral contraceptives. At the Lintas advertising agency, we started work with great caution, for two reasons. First, we had had problems in the past when the government changed or when ministers changed their attitudes. For example, an activity such as a radio advertising campaign for contraceptives might have been approved, be in operation, and be well received by the public. Then a new minister might be appointed who had problems in talking about condoms, and we would be told to slow down or stop the campaign.

The second reason was that we could not assume that we could start with the public where we had left off some five or six years previously; we had to move cautiously, step by step.

---
[a] Managing Director, Lintas Ghana Ltd, Accra, Ghana.

We therefore started with a small amount of advertising in the press and some at points of sale. One of the condom brand names had been used previously, so we used the slogan, "Your favourite Panther condoms are back". Next we moved into radio and television and it was at that stage that we ran into trouble. One of the national newspapers was against family planning, regarding it as an imperialist plot, the Western nations wanting to control our population for their own reasons rather than for ours. This newspaper refused to accept any advertising or carry editorials on family planning.

One morning the front page of the paper carried an announcement that advertising of contraceptives was banned. The paper claimed that the Government had banned radio, television, and other mass media from carrying any advertisements for contraceptives, especially condoms. For a year we tried to get the Government to change its mind and reverse its policy—a policy we were never able to examine because we were never able to obtain a document in which it was stated. But by that time the press had taken the ban to be a fact. It was a major issue; we lobbied members of the Government, asking why the ban had been decreed, what mistakes we had made, and whether the ban would be lifted if we were more careful.

While the ban against advertising contraceptives was still in effect, the Campaign Against AIDS Foundation was established. This was a private foundation which brought together people from the private sector and senior officials who could raise funds; the Minister of Health and a very senior member of the Government were at the Foundation's inauguration. Inevitably, the following question was raised: since use of condoms is considered to be one of the ways of combating AIDS, how could anything positive be done if we could not talk about condoms in the mass media, much less advertise them? This caused some embarrassment. Shortly after the inauguration of the Foundation—but not necessarily because of it—the ban on contraceptive advertising was eased, advertising being permitted subject to certain conditions.

The strategy

We then presented a strategy for messages about AIDS to the Campaign Against AIDS Foundation. Our past experience in the field of family planning had shown that the first thing we had to do was persuade the Government to support the plan. This had to be done individually with every member of the Government, because orders come from individuals. There is little point in telling the public that AIDS is a major problem, if members of the Government later deny this because they have not received correct information.

Three objectives therefore had to be achieved:

● We had to convince everyone in the Government that AIDS represented a major threat to the country, that there was no vaccine or cure, and that health promotion was the only way of preventing or minimizing its spread.

● We had to persuade the decision-makers that advertising led to increased purchases of condoms. Whenever advertising was stopped, sales dropped.

● We also had to make it clear that, when the Government banned contraceptive advertising, a significant proportion of the population interpreted the ban to mean that contraceptives, especially condoms, were unsafe. Such sudden changes in policy can have very adverse results.

We decided that the best way to put across these points was by means of video.

The video

We made a video recording aimed at all the policy-makers: the Head of State, the Council, and the Cabinet; the commanders within the military forces and police; the senior principal government secretaries; the Director-General of Broadcasting; and the managing directors of the two major newspaper groups. All were powerful people, any one of whom at any time could stop the messages if they felt they were making too big an issue of AIDS.

We knew that the kind of massive campaign needed would only work if it was seen as being launched by the Government, and that the Government would have to harness all the available power and resources to make it succeed. If the campaign came from very high up, the people at a lower level who might want to stop it (for instance a district council chairman who might not want to put up a billboard in his village) could be told that it was the Head of State who had ordered it. We also had to convince the Government that under no circumstances should they stop the campaign once it had started.

We could never get a target group of this size together at one sitting in order to talk to them all. Neither did we have the resources to talk to each person individually. We could have printed a book or booklet but, given how busy people are, there was no guarantee that they would read it. However, almost all of the target group had access to video, and we know that television is a very easy way of learning, since it is seen as entertainment.

We called the video "AIDS—Need for Action Now". We found a young woman with the disease, who agreed to be interviewed. At the time she contracted HIV infection she knew very little about the disease. She thought that only girls who visited sailors in port could catch it, and as she said, "I've never been on a ship."

After three months we filmed her again. Her condition had deteriorated so much that her appearance was a very powerful statement about how bad AIDS could be. Nevertheless, in the commentary we said that we were not going to talk about the horror of the disease, but would use the example of the woman to give us hope. Our message was that few people are born with AIDS and that everyone can take action to avoid it—but only if they know what to do. The young woman, and all the other people with AIDS, had not been told about the disease. People can die from ignorance.

We had to be very careful about the language we used. We do not have many words for sexual intercourse, and the phrase "love carefully" does not specifically communicate that it is the act of penetration that exposes one to AIDS. We found it best to go step by step, starting with phrases such as "love carefully" and then becoming more explicit, explaining that by "love" we meant penetration, not just holding hands or stroking someone's head. We had to be explicit enough that people would understand that they should not make love without a condom, but not so explicit that they would reject the message.

Using the video

We had planned to produce about thirty copies of the video recording to ensure that all the key decision-makers could keep one at home for a couple of weeks. We hoped they might invite a few of their friends to view it and so produce an immediate spin-off. We intended to take the copy back after a few weeks and pass it to someone else. In the end, we did not have enough money to make the number of copies we required; we could only make a few.

Getting copies of the recording to the policy-makers proved to be quite difficult until the Deputy Secretary for Health saw the tape. Her husband was a member of the Campaign Against AIDS Foundation, which had commissioned it, so he had seen it too. She thought it sufficiently important to show it at a Cabinet meeting, and also arranged for the Head of State and other members of the Council to see it.

A short while later the Chairman of the Council of Secretaries issued a statement that the Government was concerned about AIDS and that the only approach to combating it was through health education and communication. The Government would be making resources available and wanted everyone to be involved. A short-term programme was developed, which is still in operation. We now have songs about AIDS, songs about using condoms, and mass media spots that are far franker than anything that was allowed for family planning messages. We can therefore say that to some extent the video helped us achieve our aims.

Lessons learnt

When I meet colleagues from other countries, it seems that they often have problems persuading policy-makers to allow things to happen—to allow advertising billboards to be erected, to allocate funds, and then release them. In any national campaign, the first target audience must be the policy-makers. We reached ours using a video recording, but if I had to start again I would devise a special campaign for this target group. I would also try to be much clearer about what I wanted: do we want policy-makers to grant funds, to say "bravo", or do we want more? Once we are clear about what we want, we can work out the best method of getting it.

I would then build in some continuity and a feedback mechanism. This could be done inexpensively, such as via a one-page quarterly newsletter sent to all the people who had been contacted initially, informing them of the number of new cases, how the situation is developing, what has been done and why, and what will be done next. It is not reasonable to approach policy-makers only once and expect them to be with you forever. As for continuity, it might be useful to create a library of what is being done and make it available for anyone in the government to see at any time.

i:3343786